About *FERTILITY BUSINESS*

"A thorough and insightful self-help book focusing on the most essential fertility questions, Anne C. Belanger's writing is simple and informative, giving this book a wider appeal among readers who lack prior awareness of issues related to fertility. This knowledgeable resource book offers readers practical tips, advice, and gives hope to people as they embark on their fertility journey. I highly recommend Fertility Business to those couples who are planning fertility procedures and want to learn more about the fertility industry."

-   Zahid Sheikh,

"Anne C. Belanger explains how our bodies operate differently from males, yet we are expected to work within parameters constructed to accommodate them. The author tells readers about a 'superpower' as she details hormones, explores the endocrine system, and discusses the reproductive cycle to educate women so they learn to increase their output during more productive weeks. Readers who are ready to feel balanced, avoid pregnancy, and have more energy will naturally benefit from reading Fertility Business."

-   Courtnee Turner Hoyle,

"The book provides insights into leveraging fertility knowledge for strategic decision-making, maintaining gut health, harnessing the power of fertility for personal and professional success, and utilizing the Billings Ovulation Method® for fertility management. The author sets out with a clear mission to craft a book that will become a valuable resource time and again for so many women."

-   K.C. Finn,

As reviewed by Readers' Favorite

FERTILITY BUSINESS

Getting Down to Business
With the Business of Your Fertility

Anne C. Belanger

ACKNOWLEDGEMENTS

I want to express my sincere gratitude to my husband, Denis, who was the catalyst for writing this book and has lived this fertility business journey with me for all of these decades.

I am eternally grateful to God for calling us on this journey of natural fertility management with the Billings Ovulation Method® through the instruction of my sister-in-law, Ruth, who, together with my brother, Jake, gave witness to the inherent beauty and design of the Billings Method™, along with the witness of several of my siblings and their spouses.

I am specifically grateful to Mary Dewar, who mentored me into becoming a teacher of excellence in the Billings Ovulation Method®, and to WOOMB Canada, which has graciously provided for my fertility training and accreditation.

I wish to thank my colleague and friend, Rose Heron, WOOMB Canada's Senior Teacher Trainer in the Billings Ovulation Method®, whose constant encouragement and direction 'with all things Billings' helped me navigate the final portions of this book; I am sincerely indebted to her.

I would also like to acknowledge the steadfast support and friendship of Sue Fryer and the expert contributions of Joel Brind, professor-emeritus of endocrinology and biology at CUNY, and the Directors of WOOMB International, Ltd.

And most assuredly, I am very appreciative of my family and friends and the many BETA readers who have devoted several hours to reviewing this manuscript for me. I am also very grateful to Tanya and her publishing team, without whom I would not have been able to accomplish so much.

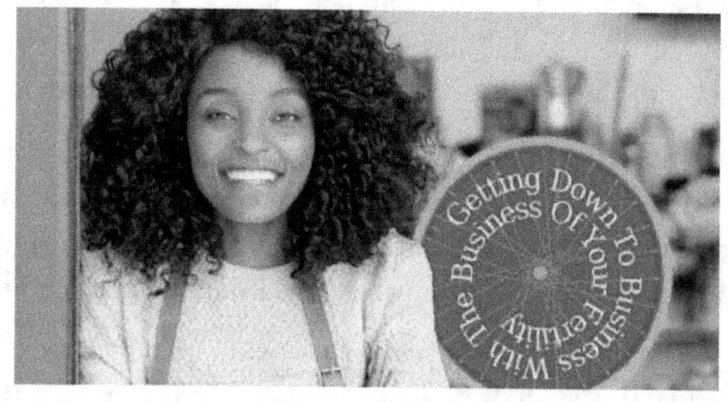

https://www.patreon.com/annecbelanger

CONTENTS

INTRODUCTION

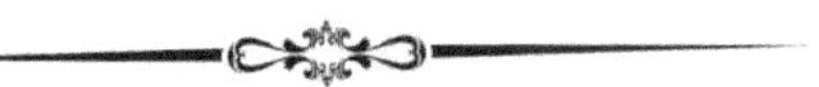

As women, we become acutely aware from a very young age that our bodies are wired differently from our male counterparts. Menstrual cramps, mood swings, waves of fatigue, and careful tracking of our cycle so that we don't get caught off-guard all contribute to heightened anxiety and additional energy to not just fit in with the world but keep up with it.

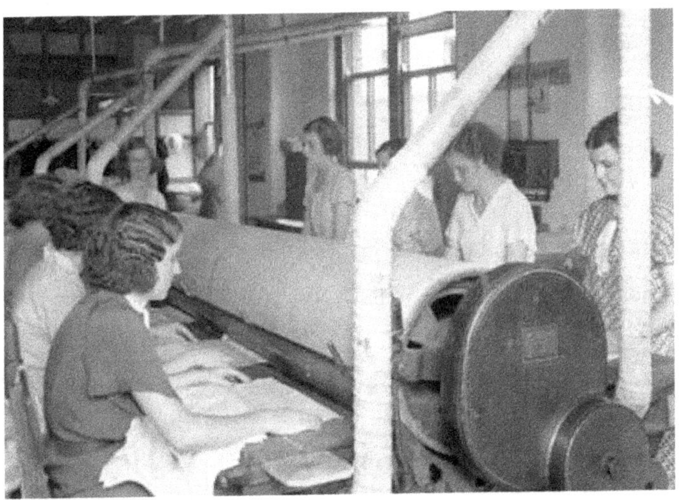

With many young girls starting their period as young as ten years old, women are pressured to accept societal norms that dictate women should conform to a system that is not well suited to them or geared in their favor at all (van der Spoel et al., 2021). One of the most significant issues women face today is the constant need to work against their natural cycles to be compatible with or work harmoniously within society. The irony that modern society deems women to be hormonal, hysterical, and irrational while still expecting them to excel at their work and, all the while, labeling them as the "weaker sex" is palatable.

Men have a 24-hour hormone cycle, and testosterone, one of the most dominant and vital male hormones, is at its peak first thing in the morning. As the day wears on, testosterone levels begin to lower slightly. Once these testosterone levels are at their lowest, tiredness sets in, just in time to go to bed, recover, and start the next day (Straftis and Gray, 2019).

When we analyze the average school, college, or workday, it is all set up to fit within a 24-hour cycle, in tune with the male hormone system. This routine suited men's school and work schedules and women's occupations of staying home and accomplishing the family's needs. So, working women are expected to conform to a routine established to work for men.

Women's involvement in society in advocating for equal rights has progressed over 180 years from when they weren't deemed to be "persons," which meant they had no say in the development or maintenance of a daily working system. It was only in 1919, during the height of World War I, when women had to move into the workplace because of the war effort, that they were legally called people once more (Silkin, 2021).

In stark contrast to the male hormone cycle, the female body works on a 23-to-35-day hormonal cycle. During this time, hormone levels rise and fall, profoundly affecting emotions, psyche, energy levels, and physical strength. These female hormonal cycles happen in phases, giving boosts of energy, motivation, and positivity.

While the world has undoubtedly started talking about the natural female cycle and how this cycle affects productivity, most of these discussions revolve around menstruation and certain medical conditions of the menstrual cycle, making it difficult for women to continue with their day-to-day activities for various reasons.

As a side effect of working outside of their natural cycle and as the perceived gatekeeper of all things fertility-related, women seek to control their natural cycle. The use of hormonal birth control in the desire to prevent pregnancy and in the hopes of maximizing energy levels, as well as suppressing mood swings and other cycle-related symptoms, can further interfere with productivity.

The issue with all of this is that women go through life having to work harder to keep up with their male counterparts. When we add hormonal regulation methods and the side effects of artificial hormones, it becomes a 'damned if you do and damned if you don't' scenario. Also, working within a 24-hour cycle forces women to put aside their mental and physical health, prioritizing a system that does not favor them.

Productivity and the cycle we work within are linear and focus on masculine energy, and this made sense years ago when women were rarely seen in the workplace. However, female productivity is lunar; it is a continuous cycle that waxes and wanes, much like the moon, and when we work toward something unnatural, we can feel unsupported.

It's vitally important that we realize that we as women have the capacity to work in harmony with our bodies, but we would fare better if we could eliminate the idea of the 'man's world' construct. However, there is a profound lack of education when it comes to women's health, and most research on productivity has been done on men and then applied to women. As a result, female health continues to suffer under the weight of unreasonable expectations set by society.

Thankfully, women are becoming increasingly intuitive of the profound power they are born with if they decide to work in a natural flow with themselves. Slowly but surely, the world is awakening to just how productive women can be when this natural cycle is honored. These natural cycles and rhythmic patterns offer the most significant source of power women can tap into, allowing us to regenerate our biorhythms as nature intended.

Living, learning, and working in a man's world has taught me that women's fertility and fertility health are often shrouded in mystery and seen as complex, clandestine information best left unshared. Our ancestors knew the importance of working within the female cycle, and knowing your cycle and fertility will help you schedule your life around your power weeks, balancing them out with your more hormonal times.

As a fertility instructor teacher with the Natural Family Planning Association of Ontario (NFPAO) and a senior teacher trainer with WOOMB Canada in the Billings Ovulation Method® (BOM) of natural fertility management, with over 30 years of teaching, seminars, and workshops experience in presenting the Billings Ovulation Method®, I'm passionate about helping women tap into their natural cycles to maximize their energy and work within their strengths.

Through our involvement as representatives of WOOMB International in 2015 - 2016, and with my experience in promoting and presenting the Billings Ovulation Method® at the United Nations Headquarters (UNHQ) in New York City from 2015 -2023 and having had the opportunity to speak with health ministers at the World Health Organization (W.H.O.), the World Health Assembly (W.H.A), and the Palais des Nations in Geneva (UNOG) in 2019, and after years of developing presentation and articulacy, my husband suggested that I share this 'good news' knowledge with women and couples of the world through a book on fertility health.

My goal in writing *Fertility Business* is to help you understand that fertility and the natural female cycle are the furthest thing from some "FBI" secret and that when you have proper knowledge about your fertility, you can positively change the path of your career, relationships, home life, and even your day-to-day planning. And, if you are a man reading this book to try to understand how you can help the women in your life put their best feet forward, I applaud you, and I know you will learn valuable information to help support them.

Helping women know where they are in their menstrual cycle and why they may be experiencing various situations throughout their natural female cycles will help them better understand and prepare for any obstacles and challenges they may face throughout the reproductive years.

From receiving an unexpected invoice to surreptitiously glancing at that good-looking Uber driver a few times during your short ride or even just preparing for a work week that isn't going to be that productive, *Fertility Business* will help you navigate your cycles so that you can use your natural fertility power to succeed in life.

I realize that much of this information may be very new to many women, as it was for me when I first learned more about my reproductive organs: what they do, why they do what they do, when they do it, and how. But if you can stay with me on this journey, I will show you an interior world you may not have been able to explore up to this point. And that world is right inside you. We'll unpack everything together, and if you have questions or need more answers and explanations after reading through all that I have for you in this book, I will provide you with contact information where you can receive more support from our websites, contacts, and associations.

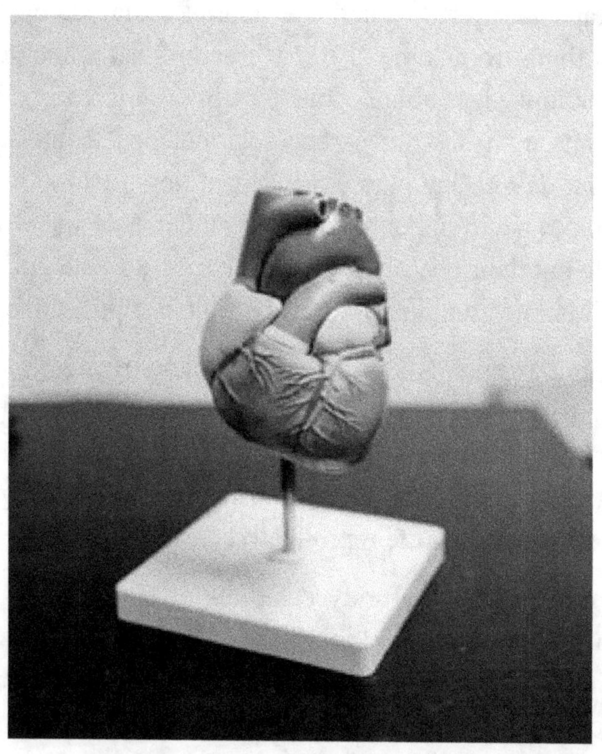

CHAPTER 1

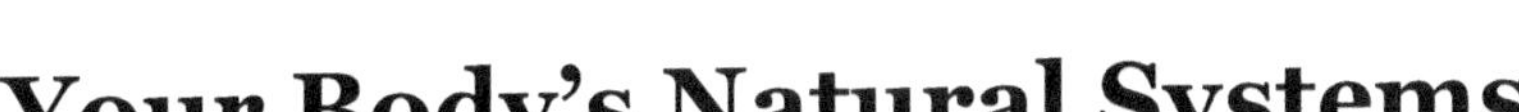

Your Body's Natural Systems

The human body is a wonderfully complex organism with 11 different organ systems. Each system is intricately interwoven, and the complex functions of each can profoundly impact mental and physical health.

Each system is assigned several essential organs and sub-systems to keep your body healthy and functioning. More amazingly, some of these systems will communicate and work closely with other systems to maintain certain functions required for survival.

When each of your body's systems is working well, and you're honoring your body's natural rhythms, your body can remain balanced and healthy. Not keeping these systems balanced or working against your natural rhythms creates a stress response, releasing hormones into your body that prepare you to 'fight for your life' or run from some perceived imminent danger.

Most people know the most common of these 11 systems that keep our heart beating and lungs breathing and remind us to eat or drink something, but our bodies are far more complex than these rudimentary but necessary functions.

These 11 systems are:

1. The circulatory system consists of the heart, blood vessels, and blood (livescience.com, 2023). This system is responsible for transporting oxygen and nutrient-rich blood to every area of the body and removing carbon dioxide and other waste.

2. The lymphatic system consists of lymph nodes, ducts, vessels, and some of the body's glands. It regulates blood pressure, plays a part in digestion, and is integral to the immune system.

3. The respiratory system consists of the lungs, respiratory tree, and trachea and is responsible for introducing oxygen to the body and expelling carbon dioxide through our bloodstream. In addition, this system regulates the body's pH balance.

4. The immune system consists of bone marrow, adenoids, tonsils, skin, lymph nodes, thymus, and spleen. This system helps the body fight against microorganisms, like viruses and bacteria, that enter the body. The immune system is incredibly complex and requires multiple organisms and healthy gut bacteria to help it function properly and keep the body safe from infection.

5. The gastrointestinal system consists of the mouth, esophagus, stomach, large and small intestines, colon, and anus. While the pancreas, gallbladder, and liver are a part of the gastrointestinal system, these organs are also a part of other systems. This system is responsible for digestion, the excretion of enzymes, the

introduction of specific vitamins and minerals, and hormone production.

6. The integumentary system comprises nail regeneration, hair follicles, nerves, and sweat glands. This system protects against external environmental threats and helps regulate body temperature.

7. The nervous system consists of the nerves that connect organs to the brain and spinal cord and ensure the body's different systems can communicate.

8. The musculoskeletal system consists of the body's ligaments, muscles, tendons, and bones and is responsible for our posture, movement, and mobility.

9. The urinary system consists of the kidneys, ureters, bladder, and urethra and removes liquid waste from the body (myclevelandclinic.org, 2023).

10. The reproductive system consists of the uterus, ovaries, and vagina in biological females and the penis and testicles in biological males. This system is responsible for reproduction and produces hormones that support and interact with the endocrine system.

11. The endocrine system consists of the ovaries, testicles, adrenal glands, hypothalamus, pancreas, parathyroid, pineal and pituitary glands, thymus, and thyroid, the glands that produce hormones in the body via the bloodstream. It is widely considered the most intricate and complicated system in the body.

Examining the endocrine system more closely is essential to understanding the natural female cycle and how hormones affect our day-to-day functioning.

An In-Depth Look at the Endocrine System

As you may know, the endocrine system comprises several glands and other organs. These glands not only produce hormones but serve to regulate almost all of the other systems in your body. Having a deeper understanding of what the endocrine system consists of and how it affects you throughout your natural reproductive cycle is empowering.

Because the endocrine system is such an integral part of almost every other system in the body, it makes sense that the hormones produced and released into the body can, and do, affect everything from your energy levels to your moods and even your appetite and ability to withstand or control pain.

The Parts of Our Endocrine System

The human endocrine system consists of three main parts.

These parts are:

- The glands produce hormones before they are released into your body.

- The hormones are chemicals that travel through your bloodstream and send messages to your organs and tissues telling them what to do.

- The cell receptors are designed to target the suitable cells in your body so that your hormone messages are correctly received.

Your endocrine system is partially controlled by one tiny organ in your brain called the hypothalamus, which bridges your nervous system and pituitary gland.

The pituitary gland in your brain produces and releases specific hormones into your bloodstream at different times of the day, during your cycles, and in response to specific environmental and internal stimulants. Once hormones are released into your bloodstream, they will travel to whatever cell they are meant for, while other cells that these hormones are not meant to target will ignore or even inhibit the messages trying to be sent.

Your endocrine system is essential in keeping all of your other systems stable, and the other organs involved in your endocrine system will monitor hormone activity so that the pituitary gland knows when to decrease or increase hormone production and release. Let's look at the different parts of your endocrine system and their specific purpose.

The Pituitary Gland

Much like the brain, the pituitary gland consists of two lobes (homework.study.com). These lobes are the anterior and posterior lobes responsible for receiving signals from the hypothalamus and for the secretion of hormones produced by the hypothalamus.

The posterior lobe receives signals from the hypothalamus and secretes the hormone that lets your kidneys know how much water should be filtered out of your blood to produce urine. This hormone, called antidiuretic hormone (ADH), is also produced by the hypothalamus, but it is secreted by the pituitary gland. In addition, the posterior lobe is responsible for the secretion of oxytocin, an essential hormone in sexual reproduction, breast milk production, and bonding with others.

The anterior lobe of the pituitary gland is responsible for the secretion of several hormones, including prolactin, somatropin, follicle-stimulating hormone (FSH), luteinizing hormone (LH), thyrotropin, and adrenocorticotropin (my.clevelandclinic.org, 2023).

Let's look at what these hormones are responsible for in the female and male body.

- Prolactin is the hormone responsible for breast milk production and the growth of mammary alveoli, a type of breast tissue. Healthy men only secret a small amount of prolactin, and usually, this secretion occurs during sexual climax. Prolactin production and secretion are also moderately higher in men with newborn babies. This evolutionary response ensures men bond with their infants (Hashemian et al., 2016).

- Somatotropin is one of the essential growth hormones produced by both women and men; it stimulates tissue and bone growth. It may seem logical that men, generally more prominent in stature and size, would produce more somatropin and growth hormones, but women have and secrete significantly higher levels of these hormones. Studies are still ongoing as to why women secrete more somatropin, but it is theorized that estrogen, a dominant female sex hormone, could be the key reason for this (Settler, 2013).

- Follicle-stimulating hormone (FSH) is the hormone responsible for egg maturity and menstrual cycle regulation in women and sperm production in men (ucsfhealth.org, 2023). FSH fluctuates in women throughout the later days of their cycles and in men during their natural 64-day sperm production cycle.

High levels of FSH in men are an indication that the testes are not working the way they should. In women, high levels of FSH indicate that the ovum in her ovaries may be diminishing, and their functions may be less adequate than expected.

- Luteinizing hormone controls estrogen and progesterone in the female body and testosterone in the male body.

- Testosterone is the male sex hormone that is responsible for male sexual development (medicalnewstoday.com, 2023). When testosterone is combined with estrogen in the female body, it assists in maintaining and growing the female body. It repairs the female reproductive cells and tissues and ensures that bone density remains healthy. Testosterone controls men's muscle mass, strength, bone mass, libido, fat distribution, and the production of sperm and even red blood cells.

- Thyrotropin (TSH) is the thyroid-stimulating hormone that stimulates the thyroid hormones and is responsible for many developmental and metabolic processes in the body.

- Adrenocorticotropin is the hormone that stimulates the production of cortisol, the hormone responsible for our stress responses, the immune system, metabolic functions, and so much more.

The Thymus

While the thymus is mainly used during childhood to help support the still-developing immune system, it becomes almost irrelevant when puberty sets in. This is because the immune system should be adequately developed, and the body's tissues should adjust to normal immune functions rather than relying heavily on the hormones secreted by the thymus.

The hormones secreted by the thymus include thymosin, which stimulates the production of white blood cells. These white blood cells are the body's soldiers that help us fight off harmful pathogens like bacteria, viruses, and cancer. Other hormones are thymopoietin and thymulin, which control brain cell growth and T cell function before puberty.

The Pineal Gland

The pineal gland is responsible for the secretion of melatonin, the hormone that keeps our sleep regular and ensures we form a sleep-wake cycle. A little-known fact about melatonin is that it is also critical in a properly functioning immune system and helps the body fight inflammation.

The Thyroid

The thyroid utilizes the iodine from our food to produce three hormones that help regulate body temperature, metabolism, mood, and calcium levels: thyroxine (T4), triiodothyronine (T3), and calcitonin (urmc.rochester.edu, 2023). Within the thyroid are four parathyroid glands. These tiny glands produce the hormone parathyroid, which also helps regulate the levels of phosphorus and calcium within the body.

The Adrenal Glands

Located above each of the kidneys, the adrenal glands consist of two regions: the medulla and the cortex (courses.lumenlearning.com, 2023). Each region is responsible for different processes and functions within the human body.

The medulla produces:

- Epinephrine, also known as adrenaline, keeps us safe when the body's fight-or-flight response is activated.

- Norepinephrine increases blood pressure, blood sugar, and heart rate to prepare the body to fight or escape danger (bodylogicmd.com, 2023).

The adrenal cortex produces:

- Estrogen and androgens, which are female and male sex hormones, respectively, and are produced in tiny portions by the adrenal cortex.

- Glucocorticoids are hormones that increase blood sugar, circulation, mood, metabolic functions, and natural sleep-wake cycles.

- Mineralocorticoids are responsible for maintaining balanced levels of potassium, salt, and water within the bloodstream.

The Pancreas

The pancreas is responsible for several bodily functions, including the secretion of two essential hormones that maintain blood sugar and glucose levels. These hormones are glucagon, which signals the liver to release glucose into the body, and insulin, which signals cells to utilize glucose for energy.

The Testes

The glands found within the male scrotum are the testes, which produce the male hormone testosterone. Testosterone has several functions, but in men, it is primarily responsible for sex drive and the production of sperm. Testosterone production occurs on a 24-hour cycle and plays a vital role in male characteristics like a deeper voice, facial hair, and much denser bones and muscles.

While women do not have as much testosterone, this hormone is still produced and secreted in the female body. Because women do not have testes, testosterone is made, in part, by the ovaries, adrenal gland, peripheral ovarian, and adrenal tissues.

The Ovaries

Biological females produce three hormones in the ovaries that are responsible for reproduction. Each of these hormones fluctuates throughout the female menstrual cycle and at varying levels depending on the woman's stage in her cycle.

These hormones are:

- Estrogen, responsible for pubic hair and breast growth in puberty, regulates the female menstrual cycle and maintains bone strength.

- Inhibin, which helps control FSH and is critical in egg maturity.

- Progesterone, necessary for sustaining a pregnancy, regulates the female menstrual cycle.

Understanding how these hormones work and the effect of their production and secretion on a woman's body is essential when trying to work within our natural rhythms.

The Endocrine System and Female Hormone Production

A properly functioning endocrine system is vital for all systems in our body. Because hormones profoundly impact our organs and moods, we must understand what hormones affect us at what points in our lives and our cycles. Each of these hormones also interacts directly with other systems in our bodies, and this will be discussed a little later in this chapter, but for now, let's look at female hormones in-depth.

Anti-Müllerian Hormone (AMH)

AMH is the female fertility and reproduction sentinel. Because women are born with a certain amount of eggs that will last throughout their fertile years, AMH begins production in utero. AMH isn't only critical to female fetuses, though, and a woman's AMH production will ensure male reproductive development is on track, too. Before the eighth week of pregnancy, all fetuses possess Müllerian female and Wolffian male ducts. At about eight weeks gestation, XY fetuses will rely on Wolffian ducts to develop testes that take over the production of AMH. The Müllerian ducts will develop into the complete female reproductive system in XX fetuses.

As women grow older, AMH production accelerates puberty, and once reproductive age is reached, AMH begins ovulation between 10 and 15 years of age. AMH levels in women indicate several great-quality egg reserves, and these levels will remain pretty consistent until a woman has reached menopause. But extremely high levels of AMH in women are usually an indication of an underlying medical condition, like polycystic ovary syndrome (PCOS).

Estrogen

Estrogen consists of three forms—estradiol, estriol, and estrone. These three forms are critical to the growth and maintenance of the female reproductive cycle, and most estrogen is produced in the ovaries. A woman's body's adrenal glands and fatty tissues have the remaining estrogen. Estrogen rises and dips twice throughout the menstrual cycle, around the mid-follicular phase or the first day of a period to ovulation and once more during the mid-luteal phase, depending on how long your natural cycle is.

Estradiol is produced by the follicle and is most prevalent in women of reproductive age. Its presence maintains oocyte health (www.news-medical.net, 2024) and the thickening of the uterus lining. As a woman ages, estradiol levels decrease. This sharp decline in estradiol in menopausal women is directly linked to bone and tissue density issues, including osteoporosis.

Estriol is secreted from the adrenal glands and fatty tissue and is more prevalent in post-menopausal women. For menopausal women, estriol is incredibly important, as it acts as a storeroom for other estrogens, converting itself to estradiol and estriol as needed.

Progesterone

A woman's body is truly remarkable, and if you need proof of this, progesterone secretion is one of the marvels of the female anatomy.

In every cycle with ovulation, a woman's body will create a temporary endocrine gland called the corpus luteum. This gland secretes progesterone, a vital hormone that sustains pregnancy and regulates the female menstrual cycle. If a woman does not become pregnant during her luteal phase, in the first few days following ovulation, the corpus luteum will stop producing progesterone and degenerate into a scar, eventually atrophying. The corpus luteum and progesterone facilitate pregnancy and regulate the hypothalamic-pituitary response to either pregnancy or the start of a new cycle and new follicular growth.

Progesterone is not the same thing as progestin (healthline.com). Progesterone is natural. Progestin, which is used in contraceptive pills and menopausal drugs, is a synthetic form of progesterone. Progesterone is not so easily absorbable into the bloodstream, so progestins were synthetically developed to mimic progesterone in the female body. Progestins increase the progesterone level in a woman's body, preventing ovulation and halting the uterine lining from thickening. Taking progestin for extended periods can be risky to a woman's health, as the risk of blood clots can increase, and the body will continually operate as though it is post-ovulatory in the luteal phase until hormone levels become balanced again.

Prolactin

Primarily responsible for breast tissue growth and milk production, prolactin is present in a woman's body even when not pregnant, although these levels are substantially lower. While most people believe you have to be pregnant to have prolactin present in your bloodstream, the truth is that this hormone is responsible for hundreds of processes within the female body. These processes include reproductive and metabolic functions, regulating fluids, the immune system, and even balancing mood.

The pituitary gland secretes prolactin, and prolactin secretion can be affected when dopamine and estrogen levels are unbalanced. The production and secretion of prolactin increase naturally during the stages of the female menstrual cycle when estrogen is high.

Human-Chorionic Gonadotropin (hCG)

The hormone hCG is mainly produced and secreted during pregnancy by the developing placenta, with small amounts also being produced in the pituitary gland, the colon, and the liver. Without hCG, a pregnancy cannot be sustained. By the end of the first trimester, hCG levels will be at their highest and decline throughout the remainder of the pregnancy. Because hCG triggers the female body to create higher levels of estrogen, progesterone, and other pregnancy hormones, it can make a woman feel incredibly ill and is often the cause of the worst early morning sickness pregnancy symptoms.

Luteinizing Hormone (LH)

LH is a follicle-stimulating hormone secreted by the anterior pituitary gland (my.clelvelandclinic.org, 2023). Both men and women produce LH, which is vital in regulating the maturing process of a woman's ovum and its release from the ovaries. As it begins to rise, it causes the follicle to produce progesterone.

LH surges once the ovum reaches maturity and plateaus at its peak (Vigil, 2012), causing the follicle to rupture and release a mature ovum (Brown, 2000). This is the process of ovulation. LH stimulates the corpus luteum's progesterone production in the menstrual cycle's final stages.

Follicle-stimulating hormone (FSH)

FSH works alongside LH to stimulate ovarian follicles and maintain estrogen within the female body. A normal puberty process requires FSH levels to begin rising, and once FSH is at its optimal level and surges, the ovum will be released, and the young woman will start menstruating again 11 – 16 days later. Children who begin puberty early usually have unnaturally high levels of FSH present in their bloodstream. Once a woman reaches menopause, FSH levels will be much higher than normal parameters. When a woman has not menstruated in a year or shown any signs of fertile cervical secretion and has these elevated FSH levels, it is usually presumed that menopause has begun.

Relaxin

Most women presume the hormone relaxin is exclusive to pregnancy. While it is true that relaxin levels will rise during pregnancy, relaxin is also present throughout the female menstrual cycle. Being designed to help ligaments and muscles relax, relaxin will steadily rise after ovulation until the end of the menstrual cycle, when levels will drop suddenly. This sudden drop in relaxin causes uterine contractions during menstruation. Your ovaries secrete Relaxin, and it is thought that the amount of this hormone in the bloodstream depends upon the amount of LH in the body.

Our hormones and where we are in our menstrual cycle profoundly affect our bodies and our minds (ncbi.nlm.nih.gov, 2023).

The Effects of the Endocrine System on the Female Body

The female endocrine system does much more than govern our sex hormones and regulate our menstrual cycle. Each hormone produced and secreted into our body will interact with other bodily systems and the natural chemicals and hormones present throughout our natural cycles.

While most of us know that certain times of the month are better than others, we often lack a deeper understanding of why our hormones affect our bodies so profoundly. Once we understand what organs and systems are affected and how they are affected, it becomes easier to understand what is happening in our bodies and to be gentle with ourselves when we need to be.

Female Sex Hormones and Your Body

Human sex hormones will directly influence many physiological and neurological functions in our bodies. The relationship between sex hormones and other bodily systems is widely studied, but most of these studies surround male sex hormones.

A deeper understanding of women's health and the effects of female hormones is slowly beginning to gain traction in scientific circles. Still, until relatively recently, women were seen as an enigma. Gender bias toward men seems to be present here, for when it comes to medicine, biomedical knowledge that is primarily favored in research conducted for men has meant that women are greatly misunderstood.

In the early 1990s, a couple of scientists recognized this enormous disparity. They began the centuries-long medical catch-up required to understand how the female hormone cycle affects women's health. Some scientists, and indeed large national institutions, have admitted that they exclude women of childbearing age because research into women is a costly affair. Still, most of these institutions will hide behind disclaimers that claim to protect potential future pregnancies.

While I recognize that the research needed is extensive and costly, the cost is based on the centuries-long research required to fully understand the female body as thoroughly as science understands the male body. The research that has been conducted and the insights received from these studies have shown that female sex hormones have a massive effect on our bodies and that working against our natural cycles is not only counter-productive but counter-intuitive, too.

Female Hormones, the Adrenal Gland, and Cortisol

The fluctuation of sex hormones can influence and affect our other systems and the production of certain chemicals in our bodies. A surge of adrenalin, for example, may create extra aggression, cause a person to withdraw, experience anxiety, or even run from perceived danger.

It makes sense that sex hormones would affect other areas of the endocrine system, but our bloodstreams transport these hormones, and this means there isn't a system that is left untouched by our hormones. The adrenal gland, located on top of each kidney, produces hormones that affect our immune system, metabolism, and response to stress or danger (endocrine.org, 2023).

Some of the more essential functions of the adrenal gland include (my.clevelandclinic.org, 2023):

- correct utilization of fats and carbohydrates

- distribution of body hair

- distribution of fat

- production of body odor

- production of cortisol

- proper cardiovascular health

- proper gastrointestinal function

- stress responses

Most of us know that the adrenal glands produce adrenaline, a natural substance that triggers the body's fight-or-flight response. Still, the adrenal glands are also responsible for the production and secretion of cortisol (ncbi.nlm.nih.gov,

2023). Cortisol is a hormone released into the bloodstream when stressed and during our menstrual cycle. Too much cortisol circulating in our bodies can cause delayed menstruation, no menstruation, or even weighty periods. This problem is because most women work against their natural cycles, causing stress. Cortisol production naturally increases and decreases throughout our cycles and will affect our mood and productivity.

During your post-menstrual-follicular phase, cortisol levels are higher during the early days of your cycle (ncbi.nlm.nih.gov, 2023). This occurs to drive other physiological processes, and because both estrogen and progesterone are relatively low during this phase, cortisol is left pretty much unchecked. As a woman approaches ovulation, the cortisol levels are reduced, and the production and secretion of progesterone and estrogen increases.

When we look at the effects of cortisol on our bodies; increased blood sugar, increased blood pressure, and decreased immunity and digestion, it becomes easier to understand premenstrual symptoms like anxiety, irritability, increased appetite, increased sense of smell, and so on.

Female Hormones and the Thyroid Gland

The thyroid regulates the body's metabolism, heart rate, and menstrual cycle. In addition, thyroid hormones have a direct effect on the ovaries (ncbi.nlm.nih.gov, 2023). While they may not directly interact with our sex hormones, they are responsible for the proteins that bind our other sex hormones to receptors throughout the body. As such, thyroid hormones, specifically thyroxine tetraiodothyronine (T4) and triiodothyronine (T3), and the release and circulation of these hormones can affect how we feel. But to understand how thyroid hormones affect us, we must first examine what they do in the female body.

T3 and T4 are proteins that " stick" our hormones to the right receptors so that our body systems function properly. T3 and T4 specifically respond to the production of estrogen. It's essential to understand that thyroid hormones do not fluctuate throughout our menstrual cycle. Still, estrogen does, and when there is insufficient estrogen present, these T3 and T4 hormones float around the body aimlessly, causing other systems to activate and try to produce estrogen.

Around ovulation, estrogen levels are at their highest, and these T3 and T4 hormones are doing what they're designed to do: binding estrogen. But when estrogen levels are lowest, toward the end of your natural cycle, and when your period begins, these T3 and T4 hormones are free flowing, with no hormones to bind to. When T3 and T4 are not serving their purpose, PMS symptoms like excess hunger, bloat, water retention, and headaches can set in.

Female Hormones and the Pituitary Gland

Hormones secreted by the pituitary gland help regulate the female menstrual cycle. Gonadotropin-releasing hormones (GnRII) stimulate the pituitary gland to produce FSH, which is accountable for stimulating ovum development and the increase in the production of estrogen. The corpus luteum, in turn, is responsible for progesterone.

About the time of ovulation, the pituitary hormones are at their highest in a woman's cycle. When pituitary hormone levels are at their peak, energy levels, sex drive, and concentration levels increase. Our mood is far better during this time, too. As the pituitary hormones begin to decrease, episodes of fatigue, constipation, water retention, and lowered sex drive can set in.

Research into the effect of female hormones on the pituitary gland is ongoing, and a lot of this research remains rooted in pituitary dysfunction and conditions like tumors.

Female Hormones and the Pancreas

The pancreas is known to be a part of the digestive and endocrine systems within our bodies, but it also serves a function in our immune system. Because the endocrine system influences almost every organ and cell in our bodies, it should make sense that the effect of female hormones on the pancreas is well-studied. Unfortunately, this isn't the case, and most studies are related to the effects of insulin and glycogen, the hormones produced by the pancreas, on the female body. More research is, however, emerging, and the impact of menstruation-related pancreatitis shows there is a massive correlation between the interaction of female hormones on the organs and other systems of the body.

All endocrine hormones released into the bloodstream affect growth, development, mood control, and metabolic and reproductive function. The hormones that control our blood sugar and how our body uses its stored energy come from the pancreas. Since the pancreas is part of our endocrine system, hormonal changes that occur naturally during the menstrual cycle will also affect hormone production by the pancreas. The most prevalent of these menstrual changes on the pancreas are changes in blood sugar levels and temporary instances of insulin resistance.

Around ovulation, when estrogen levels rise, insulin sensitivity increases, lowering blood sugar levels throughout our bodies. By the time we enter the luteal phase of our cycle, the period after ovulation which is under the influence of the corpus luteum and lasts until the start of our next period, increased progesterone production decreases insulin sensitivity. As such, blood sugar levels rise. Diabetic women, therefore, may have to battle against some pretty significant blood sugar fluctuations throughout their menstrual cycle. It is also interesting to note that higher blood sugar levels cause symptoms like fatigue, increased need to urinate, dizziness, excessive hunger, and cravings for sweet foods and drinks. Sound familiar?

Female Hormones and the Ovaries

Our ovaries function on hormones secreted by the pituitary gland and hormones produced by the corpus luteum, the ovaries, and other organs. The female body is so incredible that when the ovarian cycle is dormant because of menopause, surgery, stress, or otherwise, other organs will take over the production and secretion of estrogen. Even our hearts can produce small but significant amounts of estrogen.

During the beginning phases of the ovarian cycle, the pituitary gland produces hormones that stimulate egg maturation and release. Once an egg is released, the ovaries produce estrogen and progesterone (merckmanuals.com, 2023). Surges in FSH and LH also trigger higher testosterone production, and this can cause women to feel more energized, focused, and in flow with the world around them.

Female Hormones and the Thalamus

The thalamus is a gray matter structure that looks like an egg and is in the middle of our brains. This structure is responsible for just about all the information our bodies receive, relaying this information to different parts of the body and brain nerve fibers in our bodies and brains. The thalamus processes different internal and external sensory experiences in the brain, dictating how we consciously and subconsciously react to the messages we receive.

The thalamus is responsible for:

- relaying all sensory information except the sense of smell (homework.study.com, 2023).

- relaying all gross and fine motor movement information.

- prioritizing focus, attention, and concentration.

- assisting in thought and memory processes.

- processing sexual arousal.

The thalamus also plays a vital role in our sleep-wake cycles and interpretation of our surroundings.

Ovarian hormones have a huge role in brain function and, specifically, the brain's response to environmental stimuli, and research now shows that estrogen and progesterone affect a woman's cognitive and emotional ability (Toffoletto et al., 2014). In women, estrogen boosts memory and focus and promotes overall well-being.

At times in our cycle, when estrogen is at its lowest, the brain perceives stimuli differently, which, in turn, can affect mood. Women in menopause who have much lower estrogen levels have been shown to have higher instances of anxiety and depression, as well as perpetual brain fog and an inability to recall memories easily. In addition, estrogen levels that are manipulated or not allowed to rise and fall naturally are the leading cause of insomnia and disrupted sleep. When our bodies produce the highest estrogen levels during our cycle, we generally have much more confidence, get great sleep, and can concentrate better.

Female Sex Hormones and the Nervous System

Female sex hormones are produced throughout our bodies and are essential for a healthy body and a healthy mind, too. All hormones affect every system in our bodies, but none are as profound as the effect female sex hormones have on the nervous system.

Science reveals that the female body is more receptive and sensitive to hormonal fluctuations, and this would make sense when we think about the minuscule timeframe in which conception occurs. The effects of female sex hormones go beyond reproductive health and will also affect the skin, bones, cholesterol, and even the protection of the heart.

A couple of female hormones govern brain activity, with estrogen being one of the most prolific. Estrogen is emerging as a successful treatment for several neurological diseases, including Alzheimer's and Parkinson's diseases.

Estrogen may not have been seen as a significant contributor to mood regulation in the past. Still, limited research meant science didn't fully understand all of the effects of estrogen outside of the reproductive cycle. New research shows that estrogen boosts overall mood, and connections between brain cells increase when estrogen levels are highest. This means estrogen peaks also affect how quickly we think (Wharton et al., 2012).

Of course, estrogen is not the only female sex hormone produced in the body. Still, it's essential to break down what this hormone does to the nervous system so that we know when to capitalize on our best physiological moments. Some of the effects that female sex hormones have on the brain are an increase in the number of serotonin receptors and in serotonin itself. This directly affects how much serotonin, the happy hormone, circulates within our bodies.

Nerve protection and regeneration and cellular regeneration also happen as a result of female sex hormones. Estrogen affects cholinergic, noradrenergic, serotonergic, and dopaminergic processes, affecting our emotions and moods. Cognitive function is also directly affected by the level of estrogen circulating in our bodies. When estrogen levels increase, spatial abilities, memory, verbalizing thoughts, and fine motor skills improve substantially.

Progesterone is a hormone associated with the reproductive system, and most women know that progesterone is essential for sustaining a pregnancy and for fertility as a whole. But progesterone is also vital to cardiovascular and breast health, and because it is also classified as a neuro-steroid, it is essential to brain health and the nervous system.

Progesterone reaches the brain through two different channels, these being:

- through synthesizing progesterone from cholesterol by the brain, peripheral nervous system, cells, and spinal cord.

- through progesterone within the blood that is directly fed to the brain and the nerves.

Proper brain function relies on progesterone, as does the nervous system.

The same processes progesterone uses to protect the brain from damage and help to repair it on a cellular level also promote the repair and growth of the myelin sheath. This insulating layer forms a protective barrier around our spinal cord and brain nerves (wildflowerllc.com, 2023). A healthy myelin sheath allows messages to move quickly from our cells and nerves to our brain and back.

Clinical trials have shown that patients with acute traumatic brain injuries had a much higher chance of survival when injected with natural progesterone, and this could indicate just how much repair happens to the nervous system when progesterone levels are at optimal levels (Ahmed, 2022). These studies, which are 20 years in the making, have moved science and medicine forward light-years in treating stroke and other neurological conditions.

Brain development and cognitive function have also been shown to improve significantly when taking natural progesterone. Women who eat a diet that stimulates progesterone production are mentally sharper, experience less pain, and have better memory recollection. Because progesterone naturally metabolizes in the brain and is a neurosteroid, it also directly affects a woman's ability to self-soothe her emotions as higher levels of progesterone are released during the natural menstrual cycle.

Decreases in progesterone during the menstrual cycle trigger changes in the brain that may increase anxiety and stress and reduce our ability to self-soothe. Sleep is also positively affected by progesterone production. When progesterone levels are at their peak, it is because of this hormone's calming effect on the brain.

FSH and LH also directly affect the brain and induce cellular and chemical changes in the hypothalamus and the entire nervous system. Increased levels of FSH and LH directly correspond with increased energy levels, improved motor function, and better memory. A decrease in these two hormones toward the end of our cycle directly affects energy levels, may increase our pain sensitivity, and may even be one of the reasons for brain fog setting in.

A Word on Progestins

Progestins are not the same as natural progesterone, and they are molecularly different. They are metabolized in the body differently. Progestins do not benefit the body as a whole or the nervous system like natural progesterone does. Furthermore, progestins are known to increase anxiety, disturb sleep, and have adverse effects on the human nervous system, including canceling the positive effects of estrogen on the body.

Understanding the hormones that circulate your body, ebbing and flowing throughout your natural cycle, and having a more profound knowledge of how these hormones affect your ability to reproduce and function throughout any given cycle is vital to your physical and mental health.

Your body is an intricate organism, but we tend to complicate its processes by trying to work against them. A healthy mind wants to reside in a healthy body, and if you want to take advantage of your natural cycle and fluctuating hormones, you must honor your mind-body connection.

CHAPTER 2

The Mind-Body Connection

In the past, the mind-body connection was thought to be pseudoscience. Early science acknowledged the mind and body insofar as the body housed the mind. Still, neuroscientists have since studied the topic in greater detail, and the mind-body connection is no longer considered to be pseudoscience. The mind-body connection goes so much further than the body housing the mind. Even our thoughts, perceptions, and mindsets affect our biological functions.

I do not disregard mindset and our thoughts as critical parts of the mind-body connection. However, it is essential to acknowledge that there are actual physiological reasons we need to work to create a mind-body balance. Part of this balance is sufficient knowledge of how our bodily systems connect with our brains and vice versa. When one system is disregarded or unhealthy, it will impact another, including our minds and thoughts.

After reading Chapter 2, you will have a deeper understanding of how your hormones, and specifically maintaining and honoring a balance of your hormones, can help you maximize your productive times while taking care of yourself in the less pleasant phases of your cycle. Understanding how your systems communicate with your mind will further help you find ways you can tap into your hormonal superpowers, balancing your emotions and capitalizing on your energy when it's at its peak.

The Vagus Nerve

The vagus nerve is a cranial nerve and the longest in our body (pubmed.ncbi.nlm.nih.gov, 2023). The human body has 12 cranial nerves, each paired and located at the back of the brain. These cranial nerves send electrical signals to and from the brain to the face, chest, back, stomach, and pelvis (healthline.com, 2023).

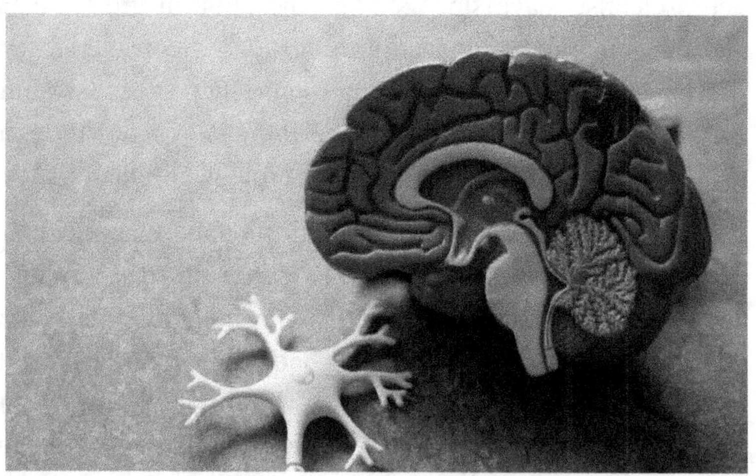

Our vagus nerve is the tenth of these twelve nerves and comes from both the left and right sides of our medulla oblongata. Eighty percent of the messages sent from the regions mentioned above go to our brain, and 20% of the messages sent from these regions occur through the vagus nerve (Mandalaneni & Rayi, 2021).

The vagus nerve is not only responsible for relaying information from our organs to our brains, though. Everything from our rest times to swallowing, our sense of touch, our immune responses, and our parasympathetic functions, to name a few, are a result of our vagus nerve.

Because of its role in the parasympathetic system, the vagus nerve is also responsible for calming our fight-or-flight response (psychologytoday.com, 2023). It is responsible for that "gut feeling" we get when something doesn't quite feel right—another pseudoscience debunked and found to be factually correct. The vagus nerve's functions are divided into somatic and visceral components. Somatic components are the sensations we feel on our skin or when our muscles respond to movement, and visceral components are the sensations our organs feel inside us.

In our thorax and abdomen, the vagus nerve is responsible for several functions, including:

- providing sensory information from the top of our throat.

- providing a small amount of the sensory information involved in taste.

- providing sensory information from our esophagus, trachea, and almost all of the digestive tract.

- providing sensory information from our lungs and heart.

- stimulation of the muscles used in swallowing and breathing, including the soft palate, pharynx, and larynx (ncbi.nlm.nih.gov, 2023).

- stimulation of the muscles, especially during resting periods.

- stimulation of the contractions needed to move food through the digestive tract, including the esophagus, stomach, and intestines.

Female Hormones and the Vagus Nerve

Our menstrual and ovulatory cycles go hand-in-hand with our hormones. Without our hormones being carefully balanced and functioning in the way they're supposed to, our cycles and, as a consequence, our bodies become stressed, which affects both our mental and physical health. These hormones also affect our nervous system and our ability to cope with anxiety and stress. This is because part of our nervous system regulates brain, digestive, and hormonal functions (my.clevelandclinic.org, 2023).

This is where things get a little more technical. The nervous system is a complete system on its own and governs many functions, but the vagus nerve forms a part of this system. If the nervous system is affected by hormone fluctuations, it makes sense that the vagus nerve would also be affected.

You may already know that stress can affect the length of your cycle, pain levels, and the flow of your period. Stress produces more cortisol, which is released into your bloodstream, creating an imbalance in your reproductive hormones.

Every hormone in your body is intricately interconnected and needs to be adequately regulated by your hypothalamus. Your hypothalamus receives messages about the hormones that must be secreted and held in your body through your vagus nerve.

Now that you know this information, it makes more sense that your hormones impact many things in your body. As you reach the end of your natural cycle, and your period is imminent, your nervous system begins working overtime to maintain a balance. This, of course, directly affects your vagus nerve, which is also forced to work overtime.

The Vagus Nerve, Your Hormones, and Heart Rate

Many external and internal stimuli, including stress, level of activity, and hormones, can affect our heart rate. If you've ever worn a device that actively monitors your heart rate, you'll notice that your heart rate and ability to recover from moments of a raised heart rate are affected by where you are in your cycle.

The interaction between your sympathetic and parasympathetic systems dictates your heart rate. Both systems rely heavily on the messages sent to the brain by the vagus nerve. Increased heart rate temporarily improves your body's response to stress, making you more resilient against stressors. When your heart rate is lower, your body becomes more vulnerable, and your stress resilience lowers, too. All of this sounds pretty straightforward, but when we begin to add additional factors into the equation, like our sex hormones, things get a little more complicated.

Estrogen and the Vagus Nerve

Vagal tone is the scientific measurement of how poorly or well the vagus nerve works at any time. The best way to measure vagal tone is to monitor heart rate, or more specifically, variability in heart rate (HRV). Estrogen increases vagal tone, which means the vagal nerve can better regulate heart rate and deal with stress responses.

When we allow our body to cycle naturally, estrogen is the dominant hormone, especially during the preovulatory phase. When it rises, our vagal tone increases, regulating our heart rate and reducing anxiety and stress responses. Estrogen levels are highest for about a workweek before ovulation, being cycle-dependent.

Progesterone and the Vagus Nerve

Progesterone has a significant calming effect on the brain, but it does the exact opposite to our vagal nerve. When progesterone levels begin to rise, the positive effect of estrogen on our vagal tone is diminished. Lower vagal tone comes with a host of nasty side effects, including lowered blood pressure, feeling faint or weak, acid reflux, increases in blood sugar levels, cravings for sugar and carbs, irregular heart rate, and feelings of anxiety or panic as heart rate remains low and the brain perceives the body to be vulnerable. For women who exercise or who work in physically or mentally demanding jobs and who have low vagal tone, recovery is much longer and much more complex as estrogen levels naturally rise and fall at different times in the cycle.

Hormonal Contraceptives and Hormone Therapy and the Vagus Nerve

Recent studies have shown that hormonal contraceptives and progestin therapy all affect the vagus nerve. As you now know, heart rate variability (HRV) is much more efficient when estrogen levels are higher, but HRV decreases as progesterone levels increase. Progestin, a manmade synthetic steroid, is not synthesized in the body in the same way as progesterone. These studies showed that women who were on hormonal medications had an increased vagal response in the first few days of using these medications, but as progestin levels accumulated in the bloodstream, their vagal response decreased significantly. This essentially placed a woman's vagal response into a permanent state of decreased response until hormone therapy and/or use was discontinued (Sims et al., 2021).

This means that when our bodies are exposed to synthetic hormones, we experience an increase in energy and recovery for a few days before slumping into a state of anxiety, bloating, water retention, and persistently low mood. Remember, progesterone calms the brain, but progestins do not, as they are neither synthesized similarly nor facilitate a natural secretion process.

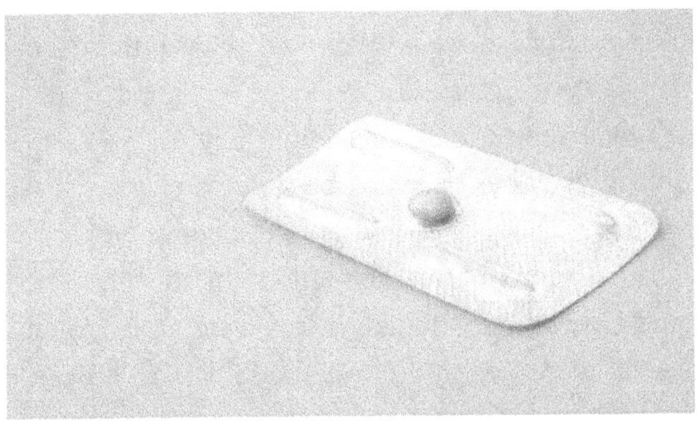

To naturally increase our HRV and work appropriately within our natural cycles, we must learn how to activate our other parasympathetic responses through our lifestyles and behaviors. Significant behaviors like sleep hygiene, eating foods rich in natural amino acids, and using mindfulness and breathwork are all excellent ways to gain a bit more control over our vagal responses. While all of these behaviors are immensely effective in improving our vagal response, one other great habit is overlooked: the effect of our diet on our vagus nerve and our brain through the gut-brain axis (northernpaincentre.com.au, 2023).

Gut Health and the Brain

Medical research in the last ten years has seen substantial progress in understanding how the gut and brain are connected. While our gut communicates with our brain through the vagus nerve, what is more interesting is how this process occurs.

You may already know that your gut is home to trillions of microbiota, or bacteria, that are necessary for several processes in your body. These microbiota outnumber your cells and have evolved with humans to continue to sustain human life. Essentially, we are more bacteria than we are human beings. With that knowledge in mind, we can understand why keeping our microbiota healthy is essential. However, gut microbiota needs to be held in check, as while certain organisms hugely benefit our health, others can potentially cause more harm than good. In the past, before processed and convenience foods, it was a lot easier to ensure our gut bacteria were healthy. Now, modern food processing, frantic schedules, and the rise of preservatives and colorants have disturbed our bacteria.

Significant microbiota maintains optimal physical health and aids digestion, metabolism, and immunity, but most people don't know these organisms also affect our brains. Our body is the host to all of these microorganisms, and their location in our body also means they have a direct line to our brain via the vagus nerve. As such, these bacteria can, in a sense, manipulate the way we think, controlling everything from our cravings to our hormones and stress responses.

While research may have initially been controversial, over 20 years of deep insights tell us that a healthy gut biome ensures our brains remain healthy by synthesizing and releasing vital nutrients into the bloodstream. An unhealthy gut biome, however, can influence our brain chemistry so profoundly that it can change our behaviors, emotional responses, and even our pain perception.

The balance between growing a gut filled with beneficial bacteria versus disease-causing bacteria is not as complicated as a person would think, and unless you are suffering from a severe overgrowth, getting back on track is relatively easy. The issue comes in with how people feel as they rebalance their gut. Because gut bacteria can and do control our brains to a certain extent, you must withstand the impulses sent to your brain that tell you the harmful bacteria want to be fed to sustain their lives.

Bacteria die-off can cause lowered moods, anxiety, bloating, constipation, excess gas, headaches, water retention, cravings, and so on. Thankfully, these symptoms only last a few days and indicate that your gut bacteria is balancing itself out.

Healing Your Gut

Before healing your gut, you must understand that it takes some time to begin feeling better. Healing your gut is essential to your digestive, endocrine, and nervous systems. Most gut healing processes take around three weeks before you start feeling better, but it can take up to three months, depending on how much harmful bacteria has colonized your gut.

Another thing you need to understand is that healing your gut is not a medical term, but that doesn't mean medicine and science don't support it or acknowledge the highly damaging effects of poor gut health on overall well-being. Wellness begins in your gut, and the disruptions you experience through the foods and drinks you nourish your body with, as well as the excessive stress you put yourself under, need to be corrected for you to honor your system and cycle. Most women will dismiss gut imbalances and side effects like brain fog, moodiness, poor sleep, and low energy levels as just a part of being a woman. You're meant to feel energetic and in charge of your life most of the time. Feeling like you're perpetually fighting against your body and brain is not normal, and you have a choice in healing yourself.

Step 1: Eat Anti-Inflammatory Foods

While I don't advocate for radical diets that could harm your body, eating a diet rich in anti-inflammatory foods is not a diet; it is a lifestyle that will help support your gut and balance the microbiota in your body. The list of anti-inflammatory foods is extensive; most contain vitamins, minerals, and antioxidants (jackiesilvernutrition.com, 2023).

When eating an anti-inflammatory diet, it's a good idea to eliminate things that cause inflammation, like processed sugars and grains, anything with unhealthy fats or oils, foods

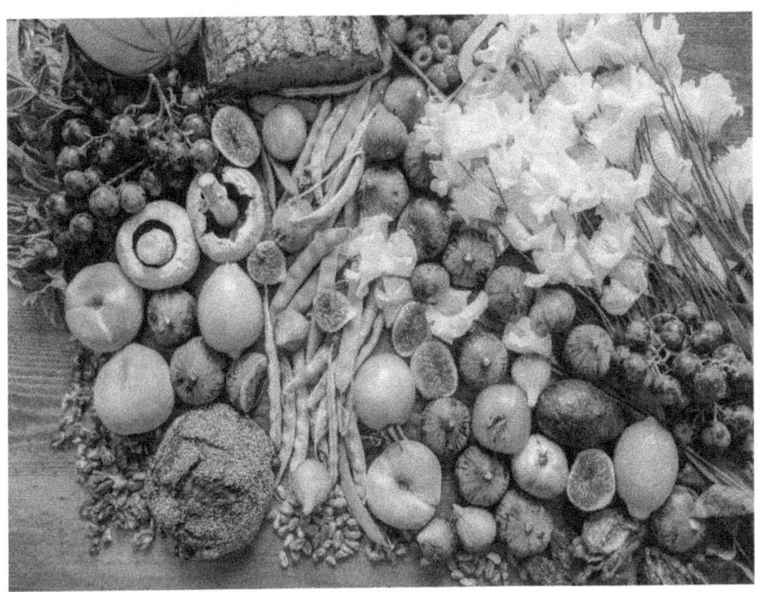

laden with preservatives, chips, crackers, and other processed foods.

Wait before you panic: I'm not suggesting you need to live a life with no joy or taste; it's just about swapping out the convenience foods with a list of ingredients most of us can't pronounce for healthy alternatives. For example, instead of eating white bread, opt for the sourdough kind. Or, instead of eating a handful of jellybeans for a snack, choose blueberries or cherries. With some research and food prep, eating an anti-inflammatory diet is very easy and will ultimately cost you the same as all those unhealthy foods you put into your body.

Step 2: Supplement With Probiotics and Nourish With Prebiotics

Probiotics don't necessarily recolonize your gut, but they already support the good bacteria in your microbiome. Therefore, probiotics support gut healing but, more importantly, nourish your good bacteria with the right foods to help recolonize. These foods are called prebiotics.

Prebiotic foods that support the growth of your good bacteria include those available when eating an anti-inflammatory diet. Natural probiotic foods include fermented foods like yogurt, kefir, sauerkraut, and brine-pickled vegetables. Prebiotic foods include apples, whole oats, garlic, onion, and bananas (businessinsider.com, 2023). Eating a diet that is rich in variety and seasonal will ensure you are nourishing your body's natural healthy bacteria in the way nature intended. Probiotic supplements are readily available to help support your new, healthy way of life if various fruits and vegetables are unavailable.

Step 3: Drink Water

I know, I know… There are a lot of people who don't like water, but it is essential to your health and your gut. Your body needs two liters, or 67 ounces, of water daily. I try to drink 125 ounces of pure water every day. I love pure water, just like I love black coffee. But if you don't enjoy the taste of water, try adding fruit to infuse it and add some flavor.

Water is vital in helping your body eliminate toxins and encourage your natural digestive processes. Keeping hydrated is also critical to producing the mucosa, the lining of your digestive tract. Avoid sugary drinks, including commercially produced fruit juices, usually laden with added sugars. Kiwi fruit is an excellent addition to your water consumption. It nourishes your body with vitamin C, helps maintain digestion, and is a great prebiotic food.

Step 4: Get Moving

Exercise is important for your overall health. It lowers body fat, balances cholesterol levels, supports your immune system, and releases endorphins in your brain.

Some studies show that exercise also supports good gut bacteria growth and that getting 150 minutes of exercise a week will help you keep your digestive system moving to expel toxins from your body. I don't need to tell you that a sedentary lifestyle is not ideal for your body, so get moving.

Step 5: Try to Be Sure to Incorporate Nourishing Broths

Broths made from natural ingredients like chicken and vegetables are rich in protein, collagen, nutrients, digestive enzymes, and natural collagen. While ingesting collagen may help connective tissues and your skin, it has also been shown to be a fantastic way to ensure your digestive system remains adequately lubricated and that your good microbiota gets all the nutrients they need to thrive.

Step 6: Be Patient and Manage Your Stress

Rome wasn't built in a day, and your gut will take a little while to heal from the processed foods you've been consuming. Being patient, practicing self-care, and managing your stress will give your gut the best chance at getting better quickly. Stress can play havoc on your body's natural systems, and keeping your stress levels down while healing yourself is essential to a quick recovery and a happier, healthier life.

Remember, the bacteria in your gut can and do communicate with your brain, and once you are healthy, the good bacteria will facilitate great eating habits. The first two or three weeks may be rough, though, and as the harmful bacteria shrink down or die off, you may have some cravings and mood fluctuations. Please do your best to stay away from all the things you know are bad for you during this time, and whenever your mood gets away from you, remind yourself that it's your gut bacteria trying to influence your behavior.

Effects of Cortisol on the Mind and Body

Your body reacts to stress differently, and stress itself has different functions. Primarily, your stress response is an evolutionary response that is meant to keep you safe and protected from external threats. When managed properly, stress helps us focus and perform for a short time, allowing us to complete tasks efficiently.

In modern society, old threats like predators are rare, and most things the brain thinks are threatening are based on perception. Perception is never reality, and for modern people, the stress responses we experience have little to do with life or death and more to do with everyday tasks that are unpleasant for us.

Issues that our ancestors would classify as minor seemingly become central to us, and when we think about additional factors like our thoughts, stress can run rampant in our lives. Think about it; our ancestors would experience a stress response to hunger. This stress response would be the driving factor for them to hunt or gather so that they could eat. Conversely, you get to go to the store and select what you want to eat whenever you are hungry. You're still experiencing a stress response, but the energy created is not going anywhere, and nothing productive is happening because of the stress response. The result is you have a full-scale meltdown, or you're irritated and angry for the rest of the day because the store didn't have your milk brand.

Understanding Your Stress Responses and the Endocrine System

When we encounter a perceived threat, our hypothalamus sends signals that activate our hormones and nerves. These impulses let our adrenal glands know they need to release adrenaline and cortisol into our bloodstream so that the body can defend itself.

Adrenaline is responsible for temporary physiological changes like increased blood pressure. At the same time, cortisol is responsible for how effectively we can expend our energy through an increase in glucose released into the bloodstream. Cortisol temporarily slows functions that are not necessary during the fight-or-flight response. These functions include immune system responses and the reproductive and digestive systems. The brain also responds to cortisol, switching it to a state of fear, aggression, nervousness, or even motivation.

Both adrenaline and cortisol are meant to put our bodies into a temporary state. Still, when we are in a perpetual state of stress because we are not managing stress properly, our cortisol and adrenaline levels remain elevated. I want to clarify that our fight-or-flight response is natural and even healthy for our body, and when stress is managed correctly, the body controls and balances cortisol to function as it should.

Properly balanced cortisol helps our bodies:

- remain alert and focused.

- maintain a healthy metabolism and aid digestion.

- control blood pressure and heart rate.

- fight inflammation.

The pituitary gland regulates cortisol levels in your body and sends the signals required to adjust them. External and internal stimuli, such as stress, exercise, wake-sleep cycles, and so on, can affect cortisol levels.

Adrenaline and cortisol production should be self-limiting, meaning it should only last a short period before the body works to stabilize hormone levels again. However, when we don't manage our stress, the brain perceives it is under constant attack, and our evolutionary 'fight or flight' response remains active. This leads to an over-exposure to cortisol and other stress hormones, and almost every system in the body will be affected or disrupted by the imbalance being created.

When cortisol levels remain elevated, we can experience some nasty side effects, including:

- feelings of persistent anxiety

- delayed, absent, or heavy menstruation

- depression

- disturbances in sleep

- heart disease

- issues with digestion, like constipation or diarrhea

- muscle pain

- persistent headaches

- trouble focusing

- weight gain

Managing stress and balancing hormones are important to a healthy life and to living a happy, balanced life. Of course, stressful situations will arise throughout life; that's just how it is, but our stress response and managing stress can make a big difference to our overall well-being (mind.org.uk, 2023).

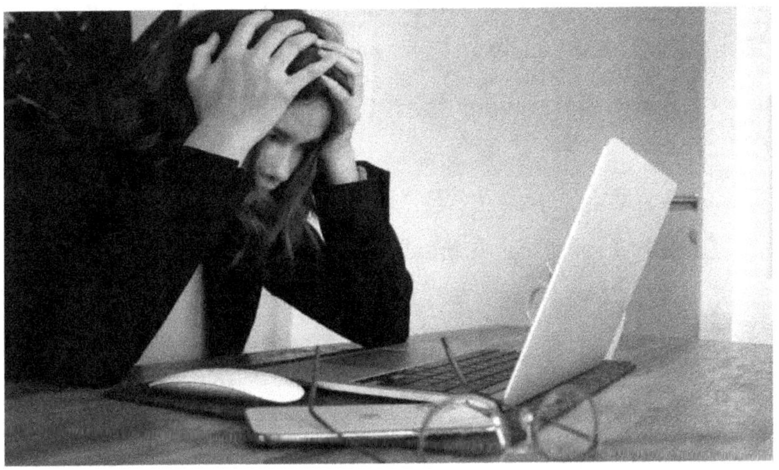

Aside from identifying the things that stress you out and tracking your natural cycle so that you can ascertain your less tolerant times, the stress management techniques listed below may help in gaining control of your stress responses:

- maintaining a healthy diet that incorporates a wide variety of fresh fruits, vegetables, whole grains, healthy fats, and proteins

- getting enough moderate-intensity exercise—150 minutes per week

- incorporating active relaxation techniques into your daily routine, including meditation, deep breathing, or massage

- incorporating mindful practices that help you stay grounded in the present; this can include journaling, gratitude practices, and affirmations

- take time to incorporate creativity into your life once a week, including listening to music, watching a movie, reading a good book, or decorating your home

- spending time with people who are good for you

- taking the time to have a sense of humor about small obstacles in your life

- volunteering at your local animal shelter or community center

- make sure you are in a routine so that you are not moving from one stressful situation to the next

- working within your cycle so that you are maximizing your most energetic times

- ensuring you are actively monitoring your stressors and finding ways to work through them

Finally, it's vitally important that you avoid unhealthy coping mechanisms when it comes to stress. Unfortunately, so many of us turn to drugs, binge eating, sugar, alcohol, and tobacco to try and cope with the stressors in our lives. These coping mechanisms only temporarily fix our stress and create additional pressure on the body's systems. In the long run, your peace of mind and adequately managing stress are far more beneficial than the temporary relief of a glass of wine.

Conditions Associated With Unbalanced Hormones

One way to think about our hormones is to equate them to a recipe. Sometimes, throwing ingredients together will produce an okay dish, but getting it right with the correct balance of flavors will make it spectacular. The same applies to your hormones. Too much of one thing, or not enough of another, can produce okay results or flop entirely, making you feel sick, stressed, and tired. But with all your hormones balanced, you become just as spectacular as the recipe metaphor.

I have already mentioned some symptoms that can happen when our hormones are imbalanced, but I will share with you a more extensive list of what may happen in your body. The reason for this is simple: you may believe your headaches are because you're stressed, but when you pair it with other symptoms, the picture becomes more apparent when it comes to hormone imbalance.

Symptoms of hormone imbalance include:

- acne
- bloating in the face, hands, and feet
- blurred vision
- Brain fog and trouble concentrating
- constipation
- decreased interest in sex
- depression, anxiety, or nervousness
- dry skin
- excessive hair growth on the body and face
- excessive sweating
- fatigue
- fluctuations in heart rate
- frequent urination
- hair loss or brittle hair

- headaches

- heavy menstruation

- hump of fat forming between the shoulder blades

- hunger

- hyperpigmentation

- infertility

- irregular menstruation

- muscle fatigue or weakness

- muscle stiffness, aches, and tenderness

- night sweats

- painful sex

- painful, swollen, and stiff joints

- sensitivity to cold and heat

- skin tags

- thirst

- unexplained weight gain or weight loss

- vaginal atrophy and dryness

- weight gain

Even though this long list may not be complete, it's a good starting point to determine whether or not your hormones are unbalanced. Sometimes, hormone imbalances can occur with or result in chronic health conditions. Ignoring symptoms that don't feel right can be devastating to your long-term health, and if you're battling through any of these symptoms, it's a good idea to speak with your health practitioner.

Hormone imbalances might be the cause of some of the conditions I have listed below, but living with these conditions will also compound and exacerbate hormone imbalances:

- Addison's disease

- congenital adrenal hyperplasia, low cortisol hormones

- Cushing's syndrome, high cortisol hormones

- diabetes insipidus

- hyper-functional thyroid nodules

- hypogonadism

- overactive thyroid, hyperthyroidism

- underactive thyroid, hypothyroidism

- thyroiditis

- type 1 and type 2 diabetes

Your mind and body are not separate, and you mustn't treat them as standalone entities. Your physical and emotional health are connected, and the impact of your hormones, how well you manage stress, your diet, and how much time you spend being active can affect your body and brain.

Your body is designed to function within a set of natural cycles, and this cycle doesn't only include your menstrual cycle. Treating your body well, adjusting unhealthy lifestyles to facilitate healthy lifestyles, and embracing creativity and mindfulness are all ways of syncing with your natural cycle and empowering your body and mind.

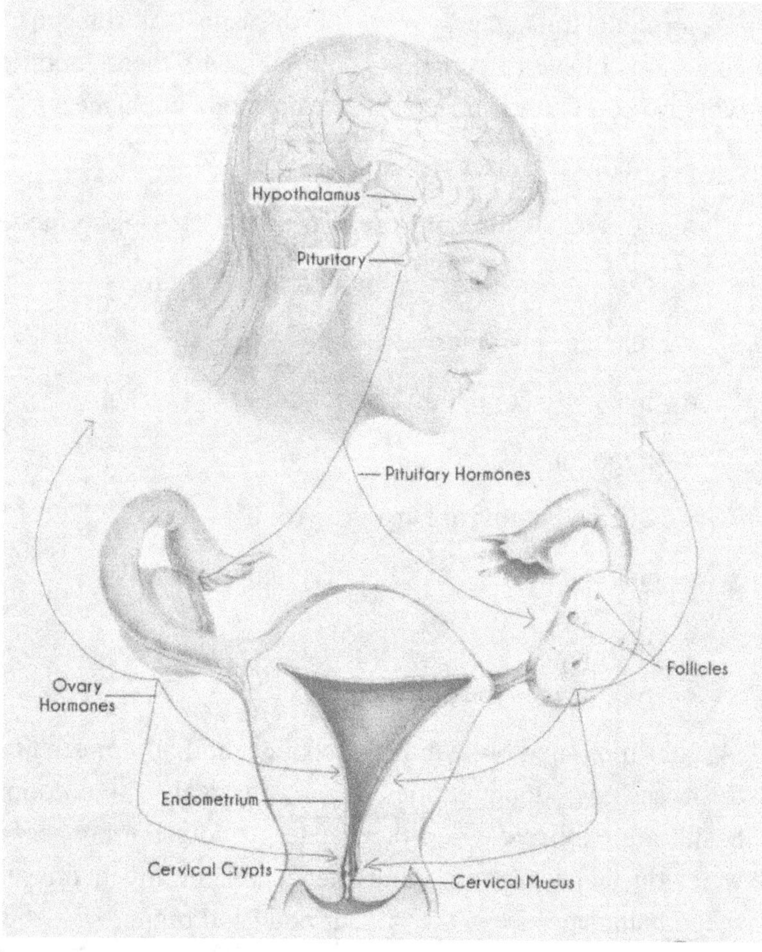

The Female Reproductive System with Hormonal Interactions For Ovulation:

_GnRH in the Hypothalamus influences the Pituitary Gland.
_The Pituitary Hormones of FSH and LH influence the Ovarian Hormones.
_The Ovarian Hormones of Estrogen and Progesterone influence the reproductive organs: the ovum in the ovary, the endometrium in the uterus, and the cervical crypts in the cervix.

Chapter 3

Understanding the Natural Cycle

Your menstrual cycle is a natural function of your body and is a complex balance of hormones designed for reproduction. Ovulation is an important part of your menstrual cycle; in fact, it is the trigger for it.

Though the first day of each menstrual cycle is considered Day 1 of the cycle, true menstruation is actually the result of the woman shedding the uterine lining from her womb because she did not conceive a child in her previous cycle. Before discussing each of the phases of your menstrual cycle in detail, it's important to understand what your menstruation cycle is and its entire sequence of events.

As a young woman enters menarche at the start of the menstruation of her reproductive years, her initial bleeding episodes may be estrogen withdrawal bleeds as her body adapts to regular cycling and full ovulatory events, when she will begin to experience true menstruation. The estrogen levels in her bloodstream, which originate from the follicles within her ovaries, cause a series of hormonal events in her brain that signal the reproductive organs to respond.

Menstruation can begin naturally as young as nine years old or as late as 16 or 18, but the average age for a girl's first period is between 11 and 13 in North America. This first period is known (or unknown) as menarche, and many cultures worldwide celebrate this occurrence in a girl's life as a rite of passage into adulthood.

At the other end of the reproductive years, a woman will experience perimenopause, often referred to as the perimenopausal transition, as her fertility declines and she enters into a state of permanent infertility. Many women will never know when their last true menstruation occurs, as they may have some bleeding episodes that occur before they enter menopause. Her final bleeding cycle is the commencement of menopause.

On average, women will usually reach menopause in their early to mid-50s, but for some, menopause will only occur in their 60s. Some women who had thought they were experiencing menopause once they were in their early 50s discover that isn't really the case, and they continue to see signs of fertility for a while.

The Menstrual Cycle Phases

A key component of infertility occurs in the pre-ovulatory phase as a woman experiences a recurring pattern of infertility that she can learn to recognize and use to avoid or achieve pregnancy. This pattern of infertility is determined by its unchanging nature and repeats itself in each cycle. It occurs before her body becomes fertile.

Another key component of the menstrual cycle is the pattern of fertility that a woman experiences as she prepares to ovulate. This pattern of fertility begins in the preovulatory phase and ends several days later in the postovulatory phase. This key component of fertility reveals itself as a changing and developing pattern of fertile secretion over four to six days, culminating in a slippery, clear, stringy discharge that then reverts to a no longer slippery secretion.

The interesting point about this key component and its pattern of fertility is that it is only established once it has completed with ovulation, providing the woman with the three symptoms of her peak of fertility. Once this key component has established itself, the woman is postovulatory, where she will remain infertile until she bleeds again.

We can learn to recognize our patterns of fertility and infertility within our menstrual cycle and use this knowledge to plan and space our families accordingly.

Our menstrual cycle is also comprised of two complementary but distinct subcycles: the ovarian and uterine (menstrual) cycles. Just as a bicycle has two wheels that cycle in tandem, so does our menstruation. These two subcycles work together, though they don't necessarily begin and end on the same day.

The uterine cycle is like the front wheel of a bicycle; it is familiar to every woman because it concludes with menstrual bleeding. As we approach ovulation, the uterine cycle exerts proliferative influences on the endometrium, the lining of the uterus. The endometrium grows fuller in preparation for ovulation. Once ovulation occurs, the endometrium remains in its secretory stage in anticipation of fertilization and implantation of the embryo.

The ovarian cycle is like the back wheel of the bicycle, and it is the subcycle that, while seemingly less noticeable, begins the whole process of menstruation and culminates in ovulation. It commences with the recruitment of follicles very early in the menstrual cycle to mature an oocyte for ovulation. In rather short menstrual cycles, this recruitment may even occur during the days preceding our menstruation (Brown, 2000). When a selection of the recruited follicles responds to elevated hormone levels in the bloodstream and the pituitary gland in the brain, they undergo a rapid growth phase toward maturity, and the subsequent ovulation of the most dominant follicle ensues. The cervix responds by creating cervical secretion that is conducive to sperm life until ovulation occurs. This secretion can keep sperm alive for several days, which we notice at the vulva.

That is a lot of information to remember: two phases, two key components, and two subcycles all connected with your fertile and infertile times. But I will simplify it for you, and you will see that once you understand why and how everything I've mentioned connects, you will have a very simple and straightforward explanation for why your body operates the way it does regarding your menstrual cycle.

The menstrual cycle is commonly referred to as having four phases: the menstrual phase, the follicular phase, the ovulatory phase, and the luteal phase (betterhealth.vic.gov.au, 2023). So, throughout many of my chapters, I will address the four phases in terms of how you may feel during each of them.

All of these occurrences are due to physiological changes brought upon by our female sex hormones, originating with the responses and demands of those within the pituitary gland within our brain. The pituitary gland within our endocrine system is directly influenced by the hypothalamus, and the function of its pituitary reproductive hormones influences the function of our ovarian hormones.

Phase One: Menstruation

As I mentioned at the start of this chapter, menstruation is the result of the woman's body releasing the endometrial lining from her uterus because she did not conceive during the time of her previous ovulation. In other words, menstruation occurs because the ovum that was released at the time of ovulation 11 – 16 days beforehand was not fertilized, so the uterus sheds the endometrium.

Menstruation is commonly called a 'period'. This nickname is both intriguing and entirely accurate. In grammatical use, a period marks the end of a sentence (prowritingaid.com, 2024). Within our menstrual cycle, our 'period' marks the end of the ovarian and uterine cycles within their phases.

However, even though menstruation is the result of ovulation, universally, the first day of a woman's menstruation is known as Day 1 because it is the most readily recognizable condition of every woman's biological reproductive cycle. The hormones produced by the ovaries during the ovarian cycle directly affect the uterine cycle. This is why, when the ovarian cycle is interrupted for any reason, the uterine cycle stops. Sometimes, women may experience bleeding that they think is their menstruation; when the cause of this bleeding is not the result of ovulation, these are not truly menstrual bleeds.

Menstruation is the process of the endometrium, the lining of your uterus, being shed following ovulation when conception has not occurred. It's important to note that you may also experience bleeding other than menstruation, which, while being the same process, occurs for other reasons. There are four common and normal reasons why a woman will experience bleeding during her menstrual cycle. The most common of them is menstruation, but we will review all of these normal occurrences of bleeding together.

The Four Normal Causes of Endometrial Bleeding

1) Menstruation is the process of endometrial shedding because hormonal support for the uterine lining has been withdrawn, as implantation of a fertilized ovum from the preceding ovulation has not occurred.
2) Withdrawal Bleeding is the process of endometrial shedding because hormonal support for the uterine lining is withdrawn without ovulation. Falling estrogen levels in the ovary cause disruption in the uterus, and instability and expulsion of the endometrium.
3) Breakthrough Bleeding is the endometrial response to the rising estrogen levels in the ovary prior to ovulation. It is often accompanied by visible signs of fertile cervical secretion before or after the bleeding episode.
4) Implantation Bleeding, which may or may not occur in each pregnancy, is a hormonal response to the embryo's implantation into the endometrium, the lining of the uterus, in the presence of spotting or bleeding to varying degrees.

During episodes of bleeding, a mixture of blood, blood cells, tissue, and secretions departs your uterus. However, menstruation is often accompanied by other tell-tale signs that alert us to the fact that we are menstruating.

These symptoms may include:

- Our acne breakouts

- bloating

- cramps

- moodiness

- lethargy

- tender breasts

These symptoms are often associated with a woman's premenstrual syndrome (PMS), as hormonal support decreases with the approach of the next menstruation.

Phase Two: The Follicular Phase

The follicular phase is the most varying length of time of your cycle (my.clevelandclinic.org, 2023). It is also known as the proliferative phase, as it coincides with the uterus' proliferative growth of the endometrium. It can be the most extended phase of your menstrual cycle, where the days following your menstruation seem to go on and on and on before the ovulatory process begins. Or, it can be relatively short, as your menstrual days may be immediately followed by days when your body is preparing to ovulate, and you are aware of fertile secretion leaving your body.

Your follicular phase is considered to begin on Day 1 of your cycle while you are still within your menstrual phase, which culminates in ovulation. As menstruation begins, your reproductive hormones are low and seemingly quiescent. Your hormones will remain in this state until the follicle-stimulating hormone in the pituitary gland in your brain becomes active again. This activity may only begin several days after the end of your menstrual bleeding. Usually, though, it begins shortly afterward. And in some cycles, it may even begin during your menstruation.

Your pituitary gland releases follicle-stimulating hormone (FSH) into your bloodstream to stimulate some immature follicles in the ovary (my.clevelandclinic.org, 2023). When these follicles are sufficiently stimulated and active, a small number of them will progress toward maturity in preparation for ovulation. However, only one of them usually reaches full maturity, while the remaining few are reabsorbed into your body.

Rising estrogen levels in the ovary cause the cervix to respond by producing cervical secretion in the cervical crypts. The body produces this cervical secretion because it is essential for sperm survival. Without the presence of this fertile cervical_secretion, sperm will die after intercourse. This characteristic of being able to keep the sperm alive is the reason why this cervical secretion is recognized as being fertile. It is at this point that your body becomes fertile.

During the maturation process of the ovum within the ovary, which usually takes 4 - 6 days, the uterine cycle begins exerting its proliferative influences upon the endometrium, the lining of the uterus, causing it to grow and thicken in preparation for fertilization. All of your reproductive organs are now responding to the rising estrogen levels.

However, the follicular phase is only fertile when accompanied by cervical secretion produced by the cervix in response to the rising estrogen levels in your body. These highly fertile secretions are necessary for sperm life and migration. Without the development and presence of this fertile secretion, ovulation can still occur, but fertility is nonexistent. Though fertility and ovulation are concurrent, they are not interchangeable. A woman may ovulate, but she won't be fertile unless cervical secretion is present to transport the sperm to the ovum.

The cervix is located at the lowest point of your uterus and functions as a valve, opening and closing at regulated intervals during your menstruation cycle. It is the organ where cervical secretion is developed for the purpose of assisting healthy sperm in fertilizing the ovum. As the estrogen levels increase in the ovary, the cervix responds to this rising level by producing highly fertile secretions that continuously change and develop as the woman approaches ovulation. The cervical crypts are cave-like chambers where sperm cells will wait until ovulation occurs. This changing cervical secretion forms a detectable pattern of fertility that you can learn and use to confirm that ovulation has indeed occurred.

The hormonal changes around the time of ovulation cause a set of symptoms, which may include:

- changes in cervical secretion that result in a slippery sensation, often with visible clear strings

- increased energy

- increased sex drive

- sharp or dull pain called Mittelschmerz, which occurs on one side of the lower abdomen for some women

Phase Three: Ovulation

The Ovulatory Phase occurs at the end of the ovum's maturation process. The mature ovum is released from the ovary and begins its trek through the fallopian tube toward the uterus. It occurs only once in the cycle, but as we know, sometimes more than one ovum is released and fertilized during that process, as evidenced in fraternal twins, triplets, etc. However, even when more than one ovum is ovulated, they all occur within 24 hours of the first ovulation, indicating that they are all part of the same ovulatory event. Ovulation is sometimes accompanied by pain, known as Mittelschmerz.

The endocrinological work and research of Professor James Brown of Australia have brought much clarity to the concept of multiple ovulations occurring within one cycle, and I have included his explanation in chapter eight. It's important to remember that occurrences with multiple ovulations all occur within the same ovulatory event, whether that be the release of two ova or more. Follicular waves of the released luteinizing hormone can occur multiple times before ovulation, but these waves do not result in multiple ovulations; they result in multiple rising and falling estrogen levels. Professor Brown noted that this research concerning ovarian activity was realized in 1953 and then more recently discussed in the research study published in 2003 (Dyer, 2003), where these waves in luteinizing hormones were considered to be indications that ovulation can occur multiple times throughout a woman's cycle. We owe a debt of gratitude to Professor Brown for all his outstanding contributions to the understanding of a woman's endocrinological system and the clarity he brought to women's reproductive health.

While the actual process of ovulation occurs over several minutes, the ovum is only viable for up to 24 hours. However, sperm can survive for 3 to 5 days in the cervical crypts when fertile cervical secretion is present. This means that a pregnancy can result following ovulation if the act of intercourse occurred while this secretion was present in the woman's body from several days beforehand or several hours afterward. This cervical secretion is necessary to achieve pregnancy because it facilitates the viability and transport of the sperm to the ovum.

As such, women can only become pregnant if they have intercourse when the cervical secretion with its fertile characteristics is present to facilitate the sperm's transport to the ovum.

Your dominant follicle, which is maturing its ovum for ovulation, begins producing more estrogen, and the pituitary gland in the brain increases the luteinizing (LH) hormone. Once LH levels are at their highest, the ovum will erupt from the follicle and enter the fallopian tube.

When ovulation occurs, sperm cells, which may be present in the cervical crypts from a previous act of intercourse, are released into the uterus. From there, they enter the fallopian tubes to locate and attempt to fertilize the ovum. Usually, one of them succeeds, and the fertilized embryo takes three to four days to travel to the uterus, where it implants into the endometrium.

Phase 4: The Luteal Phase

Once you have ovulated, you are post-ovulatory, and the Luteal Phase begins (my.clevelandclinic.org, 2023). This part of a woman's cycle is called the Luteal Phase because it is influenced by the activity of the Corpus Luteum. Corpus Luteum is a Latin term for yellow body/substance (somersetearlyscans.co.uk, 2023). The corpus luteum, formed from the luteinized granulosa and theca cells inside the follicle from which the ovum erupted in the ovary, produces progesterone and a small amount of estrogen to begin and maintain the secretory phase of the endometrium, preparing the uterine lining for implantation by the embryo.

In most cycles, ovulation will occur on the last day when a woman notices the presence of fertile cervical secretion at the vulva of her vagina before her luteal phase begins. In other cycles, ovulation may be delayed until the 1st or 2nd days of the luteal phase. And in some rare cases, ovulation may occur on the day previous to the Peak (Vigil, 2016). But in each of these circumstances, the woman's fertility is affected by the realization that the cervical secretion is no longer being developed in the cervix, and she now recognizes that the change indicates the first day of her luteal phase. Its normal and healthy length is 11-16 days.

If implantation occurs, it will take place during the first week of the luteal phase (ncbi.nlm.nih.gov, 2023). The implantation process takes three to four days, and it causes a chemical-hormonal feedback message to be sent to the pituitary gland in the brain, indicating the presence of an embryo in the endometrium and the need to sustain the pregnancy. The corpus luteum inside the follicle from which the ovum emanates will form a cyst and produce progesterone (medicalnewstoday.com, 2023). HCG stimulates the corpus luteum to produce progesterone for the first trimester, after which the mother's body will assume that responsibility. Some women will experience implantation bleeding within the first six to fourteen days of their luteal phase.

However, in the absence of the feedback message which the implantation of an embryo would have delivered to the woman's pituitary, and there is no communication between the pituitary hormones in the brain and the endometrium in the uterus, the requirement for the ovarian hormones to continue the production of estrogen and progesterone diminishes, and their hormonal support for the endometrium withdraws, resulting in the woman's next menstruation. This occurs because your brain determines that the uterus no longer needs the endometrium as the anticipated embryo has not been implanted.

Without the feedback message to the brain that an embryo needs to be supported, which would occur around the midway point of the luteal phase, the ovarian hormones of estrogen and progesterone decrease as prostaglandins are released into your bloodstream. This is because, about a week before a woman experiences her menstruation, her brain recognizes that there has been no implantation of an embryo into her endometrium, so it starts to withdraw the supporting hormones for the endometrium. This action is what causes some of the PMS symptoms some women experience during their period.

This declining progesterone, along with a surplus of estrogen toward the end of the luteal phase, is thought to cause premenstrual (PMS) symptoms (ncbi.nlm.nih.gov, 2024). The surplus estrogen may be the result of the body preparing for the next cycle. Many women will experience these PMS symptoms toward the end of their luteal phase.

Symptoms include:

- bloating
- changes in bowel movement
- changes in sleep
- fatigue
- fluctuations in mood
- headaches
- irritability
- uterus cramps

Menstrual Disruptions

One of the most common gynecological complaints that doctors receive is menstrual disruptions. There are several reasons for a disrupted menstrual cycle, ranging from hormonal imbalances to life changes and some of life's more serious illnesses.

Stress is the leading cause of menstrual disruptions. This is caused by the additional cortisol levels in the bloodstream, which can cause disruptions and imbalances in our sex hormones. Birth control pills suppress the ovulatory and menstrual functions of our cycles, but they can also disrupt our other bodily systems. Hormonal intrauterine devices (IUDs) specifically can cause menstrual disruptions. And other medications like blood thinners and steroids also directly interact with sex hormones, causing cycle disruptions.

Because the ovulatory and menstrual cycles are interconnected, dysfunction in the ovaries can cause menstrual disruptions. Ovulation dysfunction directly affects the levels of sex hormones in the body, which can cause longer cycles. Uterine polyps and fibroids, benign growths that form in the uterus, may not affect cycle length but may account for and can cause spotting between periods and heavy menstrual bleeding. Any bleeding or spotting that is not usual, normal, or accounted for should be brought to the attention of your medical professional.

Finally, perimenopause and menopause are natural phases of the female lifecycle where sex hormones begin to decline, and ovulation occurs less frequently as the reproductive hormones decrease in the pituitary gland and the ovaries. During perimenopause, the menstrual cycle becomes irregular or erratic, and lower amounts of sex hormones cause symptoms like hot flashes and night sweats (my.clevelandclinic.org, 2023). A year after a woman experiences her last menstruation bleeding, she is most likely entering menopause. The menopausal transition can last several months or years, and only when all fertile cervical secretions have completely stopped for a year and the body has adjusted to lower hormonal levels does menopause begin.

Common Menstrual Complaints and Problems

Some women breeze through life with the minor inconvenience of bleeding for a few days every 28 days, like clockwork. These women seem to have it easy with no energy dips, no cramps, bloating, or PMS. Other women will have a tough time during menstruation, and for many of us, our monthly reality consists of mood swings, food cravings, acne, and wanting to curl up on the sofa for a couple of days until the blahs go away.

The hormones in our bodies can trigger many side effects, some of which are normal, like bloating and water retention, but others that could indicate underlying issues:

- PMS: is a primarily regular occurrence in women and can affect everything from our dietary needs to how well we deal with stress. However, prolonged PMS or dramatic mood fluctuations in adult women need to be investigated further.

- Dysmenorrhea: Painful periods caused by inevitable hormone fluctuations should also be investigated further. Uterine fibroids, hormonal imbalances, and endometriosis are all possible causes of dysmenorrhea.

Women with painful periods may also experience a histamine reaction when menstruating. Apparently, this reaction coaxes the body into sneezing to dislodge the uterine lining (Proctor & Farquhar, 2006).

- Menorrhagia: heavy menstrual bleeding that occurs as a result of hormonal disruptions, uterine polyps or fibroids, or other medical conditions. When left untreated, menorrhagia can lead to anemia, extreme fatigue, and debilitating pain.

- Amenorrhea: having no period is usually an indication of stress, hormonal imbalances, pregnancy, breastfeeding, or menopause (ncbi.nlm.nih.gov, 2024). While many causes of amenorrhea may require medical intervention, a calorie deficit diet can also be the cause of an absent period (healthline.com, 2024).

Menstruation is a natural, biological process that requires your hormones to function in a specific way throughout your cycle. During menstruation, you will experience hormonal fluctuations that may affect your productivity levels, how much pain you feel, and how tired you feel. And they may even influence your eating. It is important to understand your cycle and the hormones that regulate it so that you can live in accordance with your body and nurture yourself properly.

Chapter 4

Living in Accordance with Your Hormones

Many women feel like their hormones govern every aspect of their lives; in some regard, they would be correct. But most of the unpleasantness we feel surrounding our hormones is because we're not living by them. Our menstrual cycle and the fluctuations of our hormones are critical functions for our health and well-being, not simply for our reproductive faculties.

Our societies we live in teach us to loathe our menstruation and fluctuating hormones, even telling us that we're hysterical, irrational, incredibly unreasonable, and vulnerable during specific times of our menstrual cycle. This constructed idea instills negative connotations, especially regarding our period. And, since most girls will begin menstruating before they're teenagers, this social construct is deeply ingrained in their core beliefs as they mature into young women.

When we think about it, fearing our hormones or holding them in contempt is counterproductive. I mean, can you imagine men waking up every morning feeling grungy or shameful because their testosterone levels are at their highest? Of course not! And you should not feel fearful, scandalous, or any other negative way you've been taught to feel because of your menstruation. It is, after all, a sign of health.

It wasn't too long ago when we were told that we shouldn't swim while we were menstruating because bacteria would make its way through our vagina and into our uterus. Or worse still, that our period bleeding could attract sharks if we were swimming in the ocean.

I realize that many of us have an awful time during menstruation, especially during that first day or two, and I do not dismiss the dread we experience, knowing that pain and discomfort are just around the corner. And I know that simply approaching this time in our month can make us feel anxious or fearful. But our bodies are highly attuned to our consciousness, and the issue with fearing our cycle, or any part of it, is that it compounds our stress response and can make our symptoms, like pain, far worse because of the higher cortisol levels in our bodies.

So, how do we step outside the social construct and free ourselves of the negative ideas instilled in our minds? We learn to live according to and in harmony with our cycle to maximize our hormonal power rather than fall victim to it.

A Word on Cycle Syncing

Alisa Vitti first brought up and trademarked the concept of 'cycle syncing.' But women used their cycle to their advantage centuries ago. Our ancestors believed women had a deep interior connection to the lunar cycle. And though we know that cycle lengths often vary from 23 – 35 days, it is common that many women experience an average length cycle of 28 days or so. Women of that time were in tune with their menstrual cycles and could use their hormone changes to their advantage rather than fear their menstruation or feel ashamed of it. We can do the same by monitoring and recording our natural cycles and using that knowledge in our day-to-day lives to our advantage, too.

Cycle syncing shifts your mindset from being a victim of your hormones to allowing you to understand and support your hormones to the best of your ability. Cycle syncing can work for every woman, but for those with menstrual issues, knowing what hormones are dominant or lacking can help them manage and organize their lives. Creating a life that flows with your menstrual cycle will help you avoid burnout by supporting your body's natural needs rather than living within a construct not designed with your natural cycling in mind.

Your Hormonal Framework

Your hormones will fluctuate throughout the phases of your menstrual cycle. But remember, the duration of each of these phases differs from woman to woman and cycle to cycle.

Many women are taught that a 28-day cycle is normal and that anything outside of that time frame may be abnormal. As we discussed the moon phase earlier, it may have been most common for women to have had 28-day-long cycles in the past. But our diet, environment, and immediate climate have certainly influenced how our bodies respond to the natural phases of the moon and, more importantly, how they react to their own internal environments. The challenges incumbent upon our modern-day realities influence our bodies and our cycles. Cycle lengths vary, so recording your cycle is essential to learning your normal length cycle. And now, we even understand that our 'normal length' cycles can vary within themselves; one cycle might be 29 days long, the next might be 27 days long, the following may be 30 days long, etc. (ncbi.nlm.nih.gov, 2023). Though several tools are available and promoted to help you follow your cycle, like basal body temperature thermometers and ovulation strips, being aware of the hormonal conditions and changes within your endocrine system by being conscious of them through your daily observations is the best way to achieve the most accurate information about your state of fertility each day.

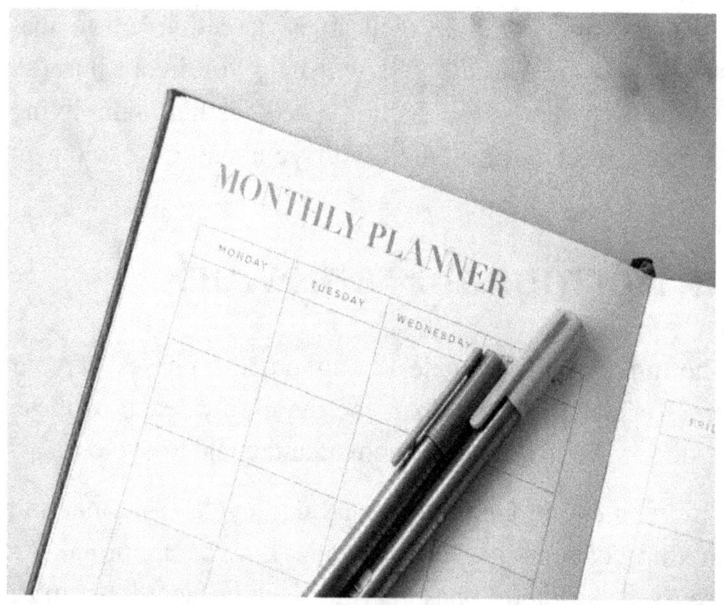

Many apps and algorithms are designed to "learn your cycle patterns" and "predict your likely future cycles." But I would only recommend apps that allow you to record your current-day observations without predicting any future conditions. Each woman is capable of learning to recognize her own patterns of fertility and infertility, and this is the information that she needs on any given day to make decisions regarding her sexual faculties. Keeping a record of menstrual cycle observations through an app or on paper also allows a woman to detect any health issues that may arise with her reproductive organs. And though it can take a few months for a woman to recognize and understand the signs and symptoms of her own menstrual cycle, learning to live in harmony with her cycle can begin today. Having patience and being patient with yourself is important, but you are not required to understand everything about your menstrual cycle before you begin to live in harmony with it.

How to Live by Your Cycle

Changing your lifestyle according to your cycle isn't new; it's been around longer than modern medicine. Instituting lifestyle changes allows you to organize your life and your health so that your bodily hormonal changes don't define your opportunities or limit you to male-suited schedules and routines.

Men and women have unique strengths, and working within your strengths will allow you to tap into your potential fully. Always remember that every person is different, and you will need to be patient with yourself and your body as you uncover what works for you during each phase of your cycle.

Journaling your menstrual cycle is a fantastic way to keep track of your hormones. On average, the luteal phase of our cycle is 11 – 16 days long. While some women will count back from the first day of their menstrual cycle to those days to see if they can recognize any ovulatory days, many circumstances could influence the menstrual cycle. The results of these influences can be misleading. Understanding how and why it is helpful to keep track of your menstrual cycles will encourage your decision to respond to the new lifestyle changes you want to incorporate.

Your Cycle and Fitness

Physical exercise is an important part of our overall health and well-being. Women are taught one of two things when growing up: either we need to push through our pain and work harder to gain adequate results, or we are too weak for specific exercises, and they are not for us. Neither of these statements is accurate; however, we need to acknowledge that certain times during our menstrual cycle can affect our energy levels.

Recording your cycle allows you to incorporate the most beneficial forms of exercise for your body during the different phases of your cycle, so that you are not fighting against yourself. I've compiled a list of activities for each phase of your menstrual cycle that you could try, but these are purely suggestions. You will know what works best for you, so experiment with them to find out which invigorates you the most.

Menstrual Phase

Lighter exercises and movements to help your body rest and recover during this lower hormonal phase are key. Trying to push through during this phase can lead to burnout, injury, and the need for a prolonged recovery, interfering with your more energetic stages. Slow and rhythmic exercises like walking, light stretching, and slow dancing can encourage better circulation and muscle relaxation. Some women will even enjoy swimming at this time, as it is gentle on the body. These are all great ways to recover from and maintain your fitness levels.

Follicular Phase

Once menstruation has ended and you're in your early follicular phase, light to moderate activity can be best. Remember, though your hormone levels will increase closer to ovulation, testosterone levels will still be lower, so intensive exercise that requires large amounts of stamina may still be challenging. Hiking, jogging, Pilates, light weightlifting, swimming, and dancing are all great options for this phase of your cycle.

Ovulatory Phase

During the days just prior to ovulation, estrogen levels are highest, and you can really maximize your workouts because your energy levels will be higher, too. This energy peak usually begins as your body prepares to ovulate and will be sustained for about a week after ovulation as your progesterone production increases and your estrogen levels elevate. If working out in a gym is your routine, you may enjoy high-intensity classes now, like kickboxing, spinning, boot-camps, and heavy weightlifting exercises.

Luteal Phase

As your body progresses into the Luteal phase, your hormone levels will remain high for about a week. Sometime around this point, your pituitary gland recognizes that the endometrial lining within your uterus is unnecessary, causing your body to prepare itself for the next menstruation. This is when you may notice that your energy levels will start to diminish. You can continue your exercise routine, though you may want to lighten it somewhat, especially as you may feel the need to slow down or stop exercising a day or two before your menses are due to begin. Follicular phase exercises are best for this period of your cycle (drbrighten.com, 2023).

Always remember to listen to your body, and keep in mind that these exercises are only guidelines. Fit, strong women or athletes-in-training, for example, may find it frustrating to slow all the way down to minimal exercise and light stretching during the less energized times of their cycles and may prefer to maintain light-to-moderate exercise throughout them. And women who are transitioning from a sedentary lifestyle to one that embraces daily fitness may not be ready for high-intensity exercise, and so on. Ultimately, it's up to you to decide what is most comfortable for you on any given day. But knowing where you're at in your menstrual cycle can give you the best sense of what to expect from your body.

Your Cycle and Nutrition

What we eat can have a profound impact on the health of our bodies. During the menstrual cycle, fluctuating hormones mean you will need different nutrition to nourish your body and help manage any menstrual symptoms you may be experiencing. Modern lifestyles often mean we eat the same foods day in and day out so that we can save ourselves time at the end of every day, but a variety of nutrients is very healthy.

Tracking your cycle can help you eliminate the guesswork of deciding what you need to eat, and meal planning will ensure you're not eating or drinking things that make your body feel worse. Before I get into the foods you should be eating, I'd like you to know that some foods can trigger hormonal imbalances. Excessive consumption of refined sugars, caffeine, and alcohol can all cause significant disruptions in your body. When reading the list below, please remember that an 'everything in moderation' attitude is what counts: though I may suggest you eat beans and legumes, it doesn't mean those are all you should eat. Look at what is on the restriction list and seek to lower your consumption of these items while incorporating hormone-friendly foods into a healthy, balanced diet. For many women, eating small portions every three to four hours will help you keep your sugar levels in check, avoid cortisol spikes, and, in turn, keep your mood stable.

Menstrual Phase

Estrogen is low during our menstrual bleeding, and these conditions can leave us feeling depleted. Your body needs iron, zinc, and magnesium during this phase, as well as vitamin C, to help the absorption of these minerals. Remember to keep your multivitamins going, as the change in our routine during this time can cause us to forget them.

Iron-rich foods like red meats, seafood, tahini, tofu, fresh herbs, flax and pumpkin seeds, spinach, and kale can be increased during this phase. Foods high in magnesium and zinc should also be increased, including chicken, legumes, sesame seeds, fish, and starchy carbs like sweet potatoes and pumpkin varieties. Cacao and dark chocolate are also great for this phase as they contain iron and calcium—just don't overdo it, and make sure you're not eating chocolate laden with sugar. Vitamin C is found in broccoli, kiwi, citrus fruits, and strawberries, but most fruits and vegetables have complementary vitamins to help absorption. For example, iron is absorbed better in the body when it is consumed with vitamin C, and spinach contains both iron and vitamin C, as well as magnesium and vitamin B6.

Active bleeding also means active dehydration, so reducing caffeine consumption and increasing your water intake is a good idea at this time. As an avid coffee consumer, I don't always follow this recommendation, but I do increase my water consumption and I would encourage you to increase your fluid consumption during your menstrual phase, too. And if you enjoy drinking herbal teas, try to opt for caffeine-free varieties (quora.com, 2023).

While fatty foods and caffeine should be limited during your menstrual phase, increasing the salt levels in your diet at this time can benefit you. Just keep moderation in mind.

Follicular Phase

Though estrogen levels are initially low, they will begin to rise as your body prepares for ovulation. Consuming foods that help you metabolize this estrogen and support your gut health is very beneficial. This can also be aided with a shift in nutrition to give your body the vitamins B and C needed, along with zinc.

Gut-supporting foods, including the prebiotic foods listed in Chapter 2 and probiotic foods, like kimchi and yogurt, are vital during this phase. Full-fat Greek yogurt, salmon, sardines, eggs, and leafy greens are all fantastic sources of vitamin B.

Some plants also contain phytoestrogens that will help support estrogen absorption and prepare your liver for ovulation later in your cycle. Foods like pumpkin and flax seeds contain lignans, a type of phytoestrogen that can be added to foods high in vitamin B and omega-3 fatty acids like salmon and kidney beans. These foods are also anti-inflammatory, which may help to reduce follicular and ovulation pain.

Ovulation

The ovulatory hormone levels are peaking now, and testosterone is also at its highest. During this phase of your cycle, it's helpful to focus on foods that support your liver, reduce inflammation, and eliminate toxins and excess estrogen from your body.

Gut health is also essential during ovulation to help eliminate toxins. Foods that are high in fiber, like asparagus, broccoli, spinach, and other crucial vitamins, will help with liver support and the excretion of any hormones that may be imbalanced. Now is an excellent time to cut out starch, opting for fermented vegetables, legumes, whole grains, nuts, and seeds instead.

Adding antioxidant-rich foods to your diet during ovulation is also a good idea. Berries and coconut are great additions to help introduce these toxin-eliminating compounds into your body. We all love colors, and your plate should contain foods that incorporate as many colors as possible during ovulation. Think red peppers, bright green vegetables, brown seeds, and vibrant fruits.

Ensure you're increasing your water consumption and reducing salt during ovulation. Keeping some salt in your diet is important for the proper absorption and use of water in your body, but make sure you're not adding too much to your foods.

Luteal Phase

The early phases of your luteal phase will require the same dietary support as ovulation, but as your body enters this phase and nears its next menstruation phase, you have different nutritional needs. Your metabolism increases during this phase, and you may become hungrier now. An increased metabolism that isn't adequately nourished will cause you to crave foods that aren't particularly healthy as you try to satiate your hunger and stabilize sugar levels.

Also, as your progesterone surges during this phase, you may feel like snacking. As such, it's important to eat satiating foods containing nutrient-dense ingredients that will help stabilize your blood sugar levels. Consuming protein with every meal during this phase will help keep you full and help in the production of serotonin. Quinoa, buckwheat, and leafy green vegetables are also great additions for increasing serotonin levels. Your body will need more vitamin B6 and magnesium during this phase, and protein-rich foods like chicken, fish, and healthy starchy vegetables all contain these nutrients.

Towards the later part of the luteal phase, slowly introduce menstruation foods into your diet. Certain foods, like alcohol, sugar, red meat, and dairy, can make PMS symptoms worse, so it may be best to save the steak and yogurt for other phases during your cycle. Always remember that everyone's dietary needs are different, and if you have special dietary needs and restrictions, make sure you are properly adhering to them and supplement them to ensure you're getting the right amount of nutrients as needed. Please feel free to discuss these recommendations with your own health practitioner and be sure to consult them about significant dietary changes.

Intimacy and Your Cycle

Menstruation is still very much a private subject, and speaking about your cycle can sometimes be met with feelings of shame. But your menstrual cycle is a necessary, natural function, and when you understand it and the hormones behind it, you can begin to embrace all of the changes your body undergoes each month throughout your reproductive years.

Women are taught that the time of menstruation is generally unhygienic. Following the pre-menstrual discomfort that many women experience before their menstruation, some women may also notice higher levels of libido once their menstruation has begun. This is not surprising, as in some menstrual cycles, the pre-ovulatory hormones may have begun to rise, causing a response in the women's estrogen levels. Though it may not be a regular occurrence for your pituitary hormones to rise during this time, it is certainly possible, and in some women, it is regular and/or fairly common. This is why, when we understand the actions of the hormones upon the cycle, we begin to recognize why we may feel the way we do. Generally, for the most part, women do not feel inclined towards intimacy during menstruation. But some women might, and I would encourage those who feel that way, to pay special attention to the days following their menstrual cycle, as those days may reveal to you that your estrogen levels are rising and your body is preparing for your next ovulation.

Menstrual Phase

As the menstrual flow impedes your ability to detect fertility, take some downtime during these days to listen to your body. Many women do not feel particularly well while the flow is heavy and only begin to feel progressively better as it lessens. Remember to nurture yourself with all the proper nutrients you need. And if you crave chocolate, remember to have dark chocolate. Dark chocolate is high in magnesium, and it inhibits the production of prostaglandins, a cause of

Dysmenorrhea, that is, cramping during menstruation. Engaging in light physical activity at this time can help ease any cramps you may experience.

Follicular Phase

During your early follicular phase, those days following menstruation before your reproductive organs prepare for ovulation, your desire for physical touch may increase. Communicating the need for hugs and holds with your significant other may be helpful to rebalance you emotionally, as sometimes we may feel we've been put through the wringer. Non-sexual touch can stabilize your equilibrium and help wake up your sex drive in gentle waves.

Ovulation

For many women, an increase in testosterone, as well as the peak of estrogen and the production of progesterone, may make you very interested in sex during this phase. This is an evolutionary response as our bodies are designed to be more inclined towards sexual intercourse and respond spontaneously to it during this time. As we become very familiar with the signs of fertility in our cycle, we will be able to use this knowledge to try to become pregnant or choose to avoid pregnancy naturally.

Luteal Phase

During the end of your luteal phase, as your body prepares for its next menses, you may feel like you're not very interested in intimacy, even before PMS sets in. Having a healthy cycle, a good diet, proper exercise, and good communication with your significant other can help you manage these days without feeling guilty for not wanting to be intimate. Your menstrual cycle governs so many facets of your life, and everything from what you eat and drink to how you exercise and manage your stress can affect your fertility and how much energy you have.

As an example of how menstrual cycle awareness can help women, a study conducted by Harvard University in which more than 17,000 women were surveyed showed just how profound small life changes can be to our bodies. Women underwent five or more very small changes to their diet, exercise, and lifestyle habits to help boost fertility and regulate their cycles. By introducing complex carbohydrates, fiber-rich fruits, vegetables, full-fat dairy, and whole grains to their diet, adding the proper types of exercise, and maximizing their cycle energy dips and highs, 80% of respondents had improved fertility and more regular cycles (Roache, 2007).

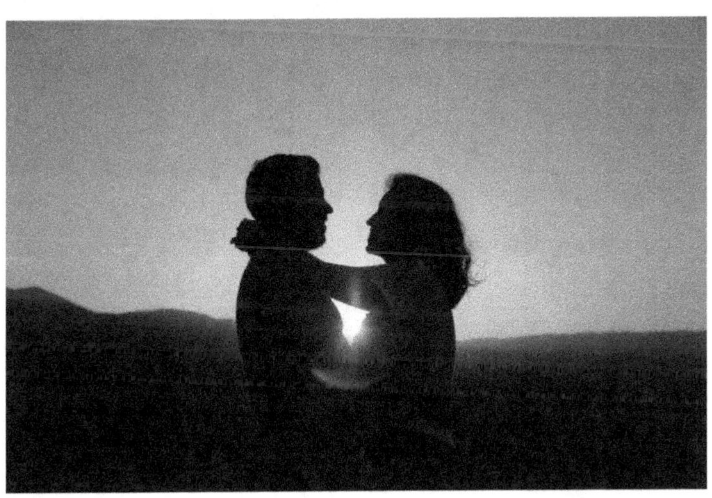

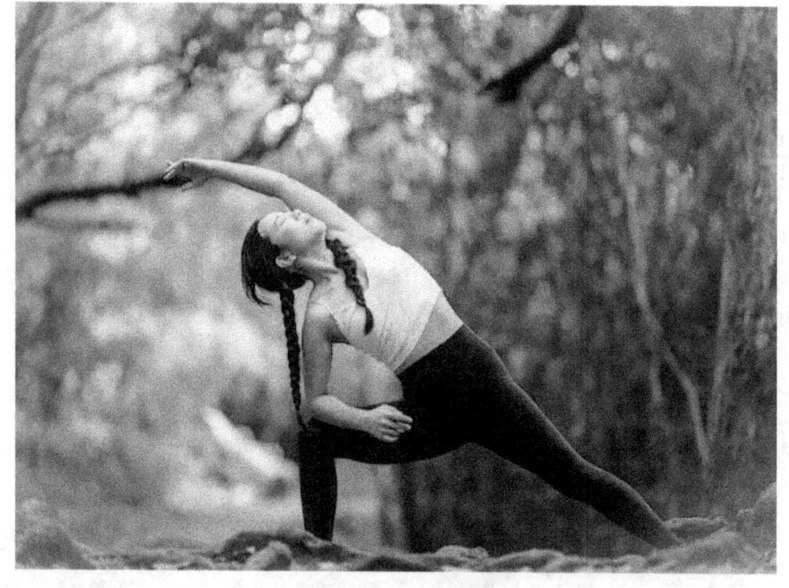

Chapter 5

Working With Your Hormones

Though women are expected to adjust to the male hormone cycle in the workplace, scheduling our lives and productive times against our bodies' natural biological rhythm is not beneficial to our mental or physical health. To fully capitalize on our hormones and become as productive as possible, we need to examine the unique patterns that emerge within our cycles and plan our days, weeks, and months accordingly. The keys to unlocking our success are our hormones, the fluctuations of focus and energy they influence throughout any given month, and learning to sync our life with our cycle.

Much of the medical research done on the female hormone cycle focuses significantly on their adverse effects, but the fact remains that estrogen and progesterone are powerfully positive neurochemicals. Many women are conditioned to believe that our reproductive hormones interfere with our ability to function rationally in the workplace, but this ideology suppresses our innate power. It would be interesting to have a thorough research study proactively conducted on women and the influences of their reproductive hormones to determine their cyclical productivity in the workplace throughout the cycle's different phases.

The fact that estrogen and progesterone are naturally present in our bodies and that we can support our cycle through diet and exercise illustrates that we can shed ourselves of this self-limiting belief and take advantage of all the benefits our natural cycle can afford us. Understanding where you are in your reproductive cycle gives you a blueprint of known patterns for your upcoming days and weeks and helps you become familiar with what the following months may reveal. This is the 'inside information' that allows you to tap into your feminine superpowers.

The benefits of working within your cycle are endless, and when instituting the right knowledge, adjusting your diet, and incorporating healthy habits into your life, you will improve your overall well-being. Aside from these obvious benefits, though, learning to live within your cycle will also:

- provide support to your fertility whether you're trying to conceive or not.

- reduce your menstrual symptoms.

- allow you to plan your day and month accordingly.

- capitalize on your energized phases to schedule meetings, lead your teams, or be the most productive in the workplace.

- work within your cycle to attain inner balance.

- plan social events and prepare for the menstrual days of your cycle.

Unraveling Your Cycle For Productivity

Most of us have learned to feel that our period is something to be dreaded. We think we are flawed and weakened by it, and our bodies are working against us with its ongoing recurrence. Some women even celebrate the secession of the menstrual years with Period Parties and Graduation Dinners. But in reality, we have been trained to work against our own bodies. The four phases of your menstrual cycle may accompany a fluctuating set of hormones, but your hormones are not something to be feared. Instead, they should be revered.

Now, I do suggest that for some women, their menstrual week may mean having to omit anything too strenuous, but as the studies in Chapter Four revealed, proper nutrition, movement, and scheduling can help to improve those symptoms. Your menstrual cycle is an infradian rhythm, which overrides your other cycles, like the circadian rhythms and daily work cycles. As with diet, exercise, and sexual intimacy, you can learn to work with your cycle when it comes to productivity and everyday tasks, work assignments, and responsibilities. Creating a life schedule that coincides with your menstrual cycle will help you understand your lower energy phases so you don't schedule that super-important meeting or deadline at the wrong time.

Menstrual Phase

That feeling of wanting to crawl under a blanket and forget about the world when your period arrives is a direct result of lower hormone levels. Consuming small portions and engaging in minimal exercise to support these low hormone levels will help you cope a little more with what you may be feeling. But fighting against fatigue and trying to be super productive is counterintuitive.

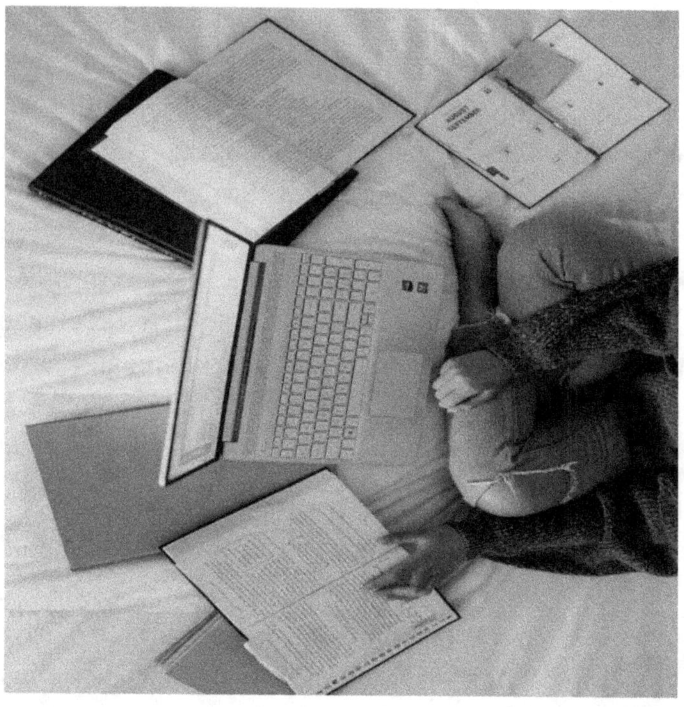

While your body may feel weaker, your brain is very 'switched on.' Your left and right brain hemispheres are firing at their prime, which means synthesizing facts, perceiving your situations, and processing your emotions and feelings are all incredibly effective during your active bleeding days. Now is the time to reflect upon any issues you may be experiencing so that you can overcome them with clarity and informed decision-making.

Be sure you are doing all the good things for your body, like practicing deep breathing techniques, light stretching, and consuming an iron-magnesium- and vitamin C-rich diet to maximize your brain power and cognitive functions. Vitamin

D is also an essential supplement for retaining a healthy immune system.

On the work front, now is the time to evaluate your performance and use your intuitive and reflective skills to strategize for the new month. Ask yourself:

- Am I currently performing in line with my own expectations and company expectations?

- Am I feeling fulfilled in my work?

- What could I improve upon?

- What has worked well for me?

Post Menstrual Follicular Phase

Once active bleeding has stopped, you move into your most creative period. Before ovulation, your reproductive hormones begin to rise steadily, preparing your body for ovulation. Creativity is sparked because of the subtle rise in estrogen as well as the production of LH and FSH, which stimulate the frontal cortex. This area of your brain is responsible for creative thought and short-term memory. The beginning of a new ovulatory cycle coincides with new beginnings for you, too, and you may find yourself curious about new information, inspired to take on new challenges, and in the mood to plan your month ahead.

Now is the time to take advantage of your creative brain by brainstorming new ideas, creating your vision board for the future, taking on and managing new projects, and event planning promotions or career changes. If you identified any challenging obstacles during your menstrual phase, now is the time to fix them. From a social point of view, you may want to meet new people or solidify relationships that may be having some issues.

Ovulatory Phase

A surge in testosterone and gonadotropin will make you feel incredibly confident during ovulation. Your powers of communication and socialization are at their highest now as your brain's verbal and social areas are firing optimally. For about four days on either side of ovulation, you may feel like getting dressed up, putting on that power playlist, and taking decisive action to make changes in your life. Now is the time to network for both social and business purposes, follow up on important decisions that have been made, tackle strategic conversations or company reviews, and negotiate any outstanding contracts.

If you have a to-do list with items you have been putting off, tap into your confidence and decision-making phase so that you can get these items ticked off the list. You may also be more receptive to feedback and collaboration during this phase. Don't forget to ask for that raise, move toward your promotion, or make career moves around this time, as your extra confidence will have you moving forward without that indecisive doubt.

Luteal Phase

As progesterone and estrogen levels rise, you may still feel energetic for the first part of your luteal phase. At this time of these rising hormones, your brain is being repaired, mental connections are being restored, and your ability to focus for longer lengths of time returns.

Physical energy may begin to decrease in the final week of your luteal phase, and you may not feel like socializing as you become more reflective and concentrated on your work. During this part of your luteal phase, you may want to take on administrative work, follow up on projects, and analyze any proposals, reviews, or feedback you received earlier in your cycle. You may even find yourself wanting to concentrate on inward-focused activities during this week leading up to your period.

Make sure you're consuming the proper nutrients by diet or supplements to help support your body at this time. If you have any loose ends you need to wrap up, accounting tasks, or even scheduling for the new month, this is a great time to do exactly that. When you follow and record your menstrual cycle and use that information as a strategic planning tool, you can maximize your time at work without subscribing to a male-dominated work cycle. You have the power to use this knowledge to capitalize on your hormone cycle, reduce your frustrations and stress levels, and succeed.

Onward and Upward for the Businesswoman in You

Women in business will know exactly how exhausting it is to try to work against their natural cycle, and it's not surprising that most women don't know how they can use their cycle to their advantage in the workplace. Tracking your cycle and understanding where you are within it can give you a clear roadmap to when your most productive weeks are and when you should shift your focus to other areas of your career, like strategizing or putting plans in place.

Working within a male-designed system doesn't mean you cannot use your own cycle to your advantage, knowing when to tap into those swells of confidence, when to be creative, when to multi-task, and when you should put your mind to problem-solving. Of course, you'll need to listen to your body in order to understand how your body works best during your cycle, but once you do listen, you'll gain a competitive advantage in your career. As an entrepreneur directing your own business or businesses, you'll know the best times to concentrate on specific aspects during your natural cyclical month.

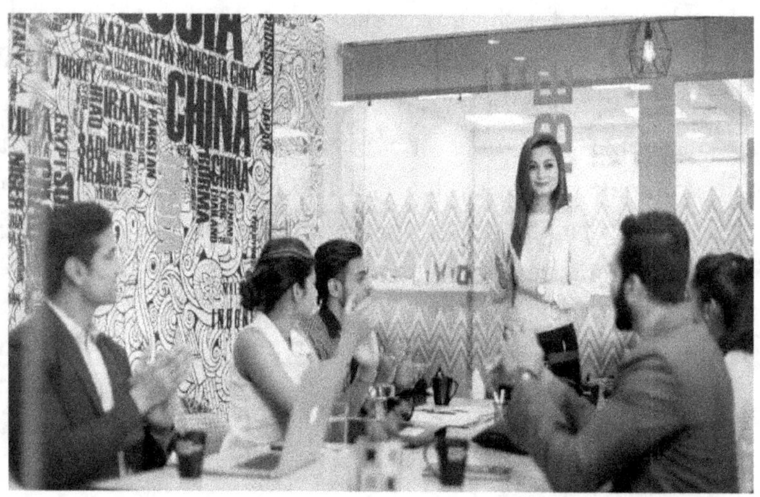

All of the information in this chapter specifically pertains to you as a working woman, and it's crucial that, as businesswomen, we can acknowledge our innate superpowers inherent within our cycles. After your active bleeding has stopped, it's an excellent time to tap into your powers of persuasion to set up new partnerships, brainstorm new ideas, and multi-task where needed. During your follicular phase, as your hormones quietly identify the subsequent ovum for ovulation, you can better inspire your teams, motivating them to take on challenging tasks or tackle new problems.

Approaching ovulation, you'll find your confidence soaring, and if you have any big deals to close or essential clients to approach, now is the time to influence them with your assertiveness and confidence. You may even find you are more articulate around ovulation. Now is an excellent time to discuss any concerns with your stakeholders and make solid plans to rectify or overcome issues you or your teams may face.

As your luteal phase settles in, solo work reigns supreme, and you may be less tolerant of collaborative projects. This doesn't mean you cannot direct your teams, but you may prefer independent tasks and be more inclined to strategize how your teams can work more efficiently. In fact, during the first week of your luteal phase, your decision-making skills will be heightened and on fire, and you will be able to clearly and concisely direct others in what is expected of them over the next week or two.

During the second week of this phase, your powers of concentration are elevated, and you can take on all of those administrative tasks you have been avoiding all month. Now is the time to do more profound research on your business goals, create detailed strategies, review staff performance, and assemble your schedule for the following month.

During your active bleeding days, it is time to reflect and, if possible, work from home. If you need to go into the office, you may want to avoid holding meetings and focus on self-reflective and repetitive tasks that don't consume too much of your energy.

When Your Cycle Reveals Signs of Stress

As with other aspects of our health, we tend to believe that we may need to see a doctor when our cycle doesn't fall within a specific set of societal or social norms. The length of menstrual cycles can vary between 23 and 35 days and still be considered normal length (kidshealth.org, 2023). Some women may experience even shorter cycles, though less commonly. If your cycle length is longer than 35 days, your ovulation may be delayed. In some circumstances, having longer cycles is normal, and by recording your cycle observations consistently, you will learn when these circumstances may occur. But if you are bleeding for more than ten days, and your periods are extremely painful or heavy, etc., something may be amiss, and you should speak to your doctor or a healthcare professional about them.

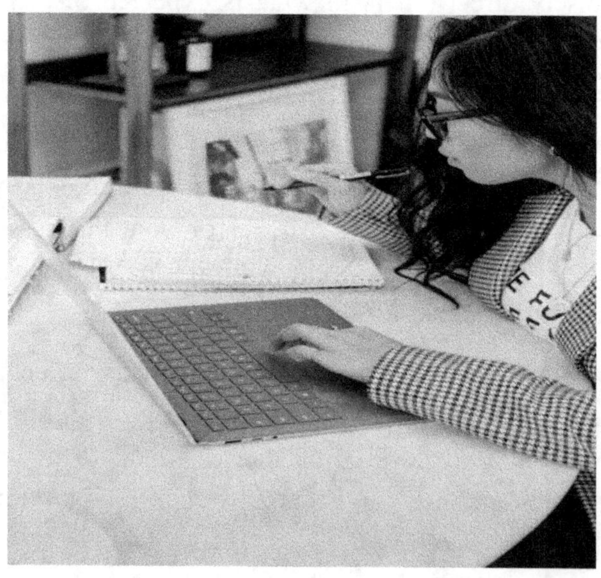

If your cycles seem relatively normal, but you are battling against severe PMS, having acne breakouts, or feeling like you're fighting with your body every step of the way, you may want to take a deeper dive into what may be affecting them.

Your hormones can affect every area of your productivity, from business to home, and your relationships and future planning. Because hormones like dopamine, endorphins, oxytocin, and serotonin production affect your menstrual cycle, your success, or at the very least, the ease of your success, relies on you listening to your body and your hormones. Many of us live with a modern diet and a relatively sedentary lifestyle, and this can affect our hormones and our gut health, leaving us to feel like we're fighting a raging war with our bodies.

As you learn to keep track of your menstrual cycle, you might find inconsistencies with the patterns you are experiencing. If that's the case, concentrating on rebalancing your hormones may also be helpful. Having imbalanced hormones is the primary cause for women to stop trying to sync their daily lives with their cycle altogether. But remember, it's not the tool of following the rhythm of your cycle that is not working for you; instead, it's applying the tool to a system that isn't working right for you — just like trying to perform at your optimum within a male workday system.

Taking the time to resolve your hormonal imbalances with the help of your doctor or health practitioner and through proper diet and exercise can help you reclaim your body as you grow confident in following your menstrual cycles. I realize I am repeating myself in encouraging a healthy diet, but what you consume genuinely makes a difference to your overall health and, ultimately, your hormone health. You don't need to be overly restrictive unless that is the advice of your doctor, but you do need to understand that absolutely everything you put into your body counts toward negative or positive nutrition.

Perhaps you are confident you're eating correctly, but you might not be considering the flavored Starbucks latte you purchased on the way to work. Something as simple as your favorite hot beverage could be filled with multiple teaspoons of sugar. To keep that in perspective, women should only consume as much as nine teaspoons of sugar daily, which means we may exceed that limit when we consume fruits, vegetables, or even ketchup with our supper if we drink a latte daily. I love good coffee, and I indulge in lattes often enough. But, as coffee is my favorite hot beverage, I decided to drink it black daily, eliminating the excess sugar and calories from my diet.

It's beneficial to be mindful of what you eat and drink throughout the day and pay attention to what you are craving so you can nourish your body correctly. Craving chocolate, for example, doesn't indicate that you want sugar or dairy but that your body may need magnesium. This mineral can also be found in spinach, brown rice, bananas, and sweet potatoes. If you feel like eating chocolate, opt for dark chocolate, which contains far less sugar. A hundred grams of milk chocolate has as much as 12 teaspoons of sugar, while dark chocolate contains about four teaspoons. Mindful eating can also help you stay in tune with your body and its natural rhythms to tap into your body's intuitive needs (weightwatchers.com, 2023).

Finally, we know the benefits of a proper sleep hygiene routine and adequate sleep quality are plentiful. Good sleep can significantly reduce cortisol levels and keep your other hormones in balance. A bedtime routine encompassing 45 minutes of no screen time is considered the best way to help you and your body relax and prepare for a whole night's sleep.

It shouldn't take long for your body to heal once you incorporate the proper steps to look after it. Please keep track of your changes and give your body time to heal. If your cycle isn't more consistent after three months, and you're still suffering through enormous energy slumps and challenging menstrual periods, you may need to seek professional help. The information you record about your cycle and its challenges will help lay the groundwork for whatever course of action you and your healthcare practitioner decide will be best.

As you can see from the information above, there are no unproductive times during your cycle. Unlike your male counterparts, you can acquire different types of productivity at various times. Your cycle can sometimes be frustrating and will not always work precisely with you. But resetting them, checking your nutrients and exercise, and ensuring you have the right expectations for yourself during the right time frames will help you fine-tune your hormonal superpowers.

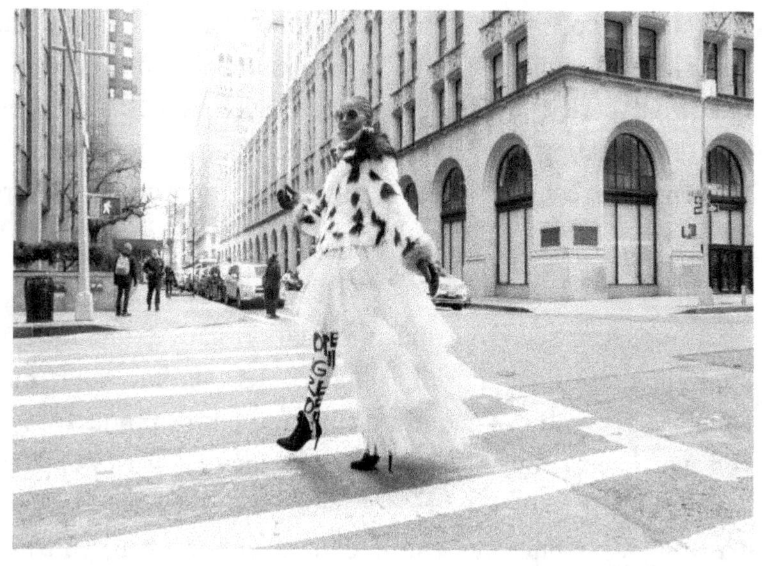

Chapter 6

Using Your Hormones as a Superpower

Before continuing our journey with this chapter, I'd like you to take a moment and reflect upon how you would feel about your menstrual cycle if you hadn't been imbued with a plethora of self-limiting beliefs. What if you knew right from the beginning of your journey into adulthood that estrogen protects your heart and brain, improves body toning, and boosts your mood? Would you have used this hormone to your benefit, or would you still be in the position of fearing your hormones and believing they're something terrible that has happened to women? Once you can shed yourself of these self-limiting beliefs and tap into the strength each of your hormones provides you, you can unlock your superpowers.

Think of your body as a puzzle. You've lived most of your life with some puzzle pieces missing, and once you understand your hormones and how they fit properly into this puzzle, you can see the bigger picture. The information laid out for you in the preceding chapters helped you find these puzzle pieces. But knowing your body and treating yourself respectfully, as you would treat your best friend, is like putting those pieces together in the right place.

Know Your Body and Shed Your Self-Limiting Beliefs

Your body and its functions are God-given and glorious. There is nothing to feel shameful about, nor should you feel anything other than positivity and love for your body. From a young age, girls are taught that our bodies are shameful. We're taught that burping, flatulence, and growing body hair are unacceptable for girls to discuss or experience in public. At the same time, however, our male counterparts cheer each other along as they attempt to burp the longest or the loudest. Think about it... bowel movements and passing gas are hilarious topics for boys and even encouraged, but for girls, this behavior is unladylike and absolutely not acceptable. We are not very good at accepting our own female body and its bodily functions.

But your body is an amazing vessel that houses your energy and your spirit. It is a part of you, and it is you. Accepting your body for what it is goes a long way toward accepting yourself for who you are. Together, each and both bring harmony to your soul. Understanding your natural cycle is vital to living a fulfilling, energetic, and vibrant life, and you can choose to reconnect with your body, shed yourself of unfavorable beliefs, and live in harmony with yourself.

The hormones that govern your cycle influence your energy levels, your ability to concentrate, and how mindful you are at any given time within a month. Tracking your cycle and getting to know your body will allow you to tap into your superpowers and listen to what your body needs.

Young boys learn to honor their bodies and take care of them from early on, taking advantage of their hormones, even without knowing it. Think about it: most men will hit the gym or start their exercise routine first thing in the morning, finish most of their work early, and reserve evenings to take it easy with hobbies, pastimes, etc. Men may not fully understand why they follow this pattern, but most will tell you their routines are in place because they 'just feel right.'

Instead of expecting yourself to get up and push yourself to perform at your best first thing in the morning, day in and day out, you should know that this is true for you as well. Doing what 'just feels right' for your body is critical to your physical and mental well-being. As you reflect on your daily schedule, think about how many windows of opportunity you may have missed by trying to live your life within a male-dominated system.

Each phase of your cycle is unique, and aligning yourself with these phases every month resembles the four seasons we experience yearly. Always remember that the length of a normal cycle varies from woman to woman; that's why you observe and record your own cycle (nitubajekal.com, 2023). Additionally, every phase of your cycle has rhythmic changes, just like the seasons.

Ways to Reconnect With Your Body

Getting to know your body is often associated with sexual connotations, but reconnecting with your body extends to so much more than your sexuality and your reproductive system. For women, a frantic schedule, limiting beliefs, and a media that teaches us our bodies are shameful unless they look and perform in a certain way constantly shape us, causing us to become detached from ourselves at a very early age. Learning to intuitively get in touch with your body and listen to its needs will help you become the person you were created to be. Forming a deep connection with your body enables you to understand how truly magnificent and unique it is so you can learn to make the right decisions for your health and well-being as often as possible.

A lot of our disconnection from our bodies derives from when we were girls when we were taught to keep our hands, faces, and feet clean, cover up our bodies, and shave off excess hair when it appeared in unsightly places. Meanwhile, boys were encouraged to play outside, often going barefoot and getting dirty at times. Nakedness is described as a 'man thing,' and pubic and other bodily hair are viewed as their rite of passage into adulthood.

Women are launched into adulthood in the most paradoxical ways, where we must act like ladies but hide our natural adult functions and distinguishing markers, like our menstrual cycle symptoms, evolving body, and resulting body hair. But there is good news; you can redefine those reasons that may have detached you from your body and made you lose that intuitive, intimate connection. And this reconnection can begin with simple practices you can do every day.

Reestablish Your Body's Connection to Earth

Tapping into your inner child, walking barefoot often, touching trees, eating plant-based foods, and feeling the sun and breeze on your face are fantastic ways to become intimate with your body again. Your corporal body is natural and thrives on nature to remain healthy.

Plant-based foods are rich in the antioxidants, vitamins, and minerals your body needs to flourish and feed your gut bacteria with nutrient-dense prebiotics. The sun helps your body synthesize vitamin D to use the calcium and phosphorus in your body correctly. Walking barefoot and touching our nature-based surroundings exposes our bodies to bacteria in micro-doses, improving the efficiency of our immune system and lowering allergic reactions.

Explore Your Body Mindfully

Throughout our lives, women are subjected to ideal body types and standards. Everything from the toys we play with to the media we visually and even audibly consume bombards us with what we should look like, according to society. As a result, we associate our bodies with sight more than any other sense. We begin navigating who we are with our eyes and shy away from using our different senses as strongly.

Exploring your body mindfully through sensation, hearing, smell, and even taste will allow you to truly get in touch with who you are. Try noticing how your skin feels as you apply lotion or essential oils to it, and pay attention to the scents these additions have. How does your body react to certain fabrics and clothes? Sometimes, we have favorite pieces of clothing, but we haven't taken the time to analyze why they are our favorites. It could be how they fit us, the type of fabric, or their weight or shape. Take some time to discover them and be mindful of why we love them. This mindfulness helps us to love ourselves, too.

Listen to the internal sounds that your body makes. Your heartbeat and breath are not very obvious but can be detected if you pay attention. The sound of your stomach gurgling or your teeth grinding or chewing is more pronounced, and we hear them frequently, but we don't necessarily realize just how familiar we are with them until something different arises. What does it sound like when your hairbrush moves through your hair or your clothes slide onto your body? Listen to the sounds of your body intentionally.

Everyone has a natural body scent, and though we may not pay much attention to it, we can become conscious of it when we choose to notice it. Sometimes, we encounter internal body smells that are normal and healthy, while at other times, they alert us to a concern that may need some specific attention to alleviate.

Choose to prepare your food and drinks mindfully, noticing each item's sounds, colors, aromas, and feel as you prepare them to nourish your body. Consider what each flavor brings to your senses as you chew and swallow, even detecting if you can feel your food as it travels down to your stomach. I thoroughly enjoy sipping black coffee and feeling it warm my insides as it descends into my stomach. I'm easily chilled and most often running on adrenaline, so indulging in a cup of warm black coffee boosts my spirit, my psyche, and my body.

Engage as many of your senses as you can at least twice a day until you feel comfortably familiar with your body. This will help you move away from relying solely on visual representation and back into a complete exploration of yourself and your well-being.

Take the Time to Love the Parts of You That Society Tells You Not To

Every part of your body is something to love and appreciate, but we were taught not to like it at some stage. Take the time to appreciate all of your body, even the parts you don't like, and express love for it. That bump at the bottom of your stomach houses your uterus and makes you uniquely female; that excess cellulite that you'd rather not have is a normal part of being a woman; your stretch marks are a badge of honor (nutritionnowcounseling.com, 2023). There is no part of you that you should not love and appreciate, so don't let society dictate to you that your body is unlovable.

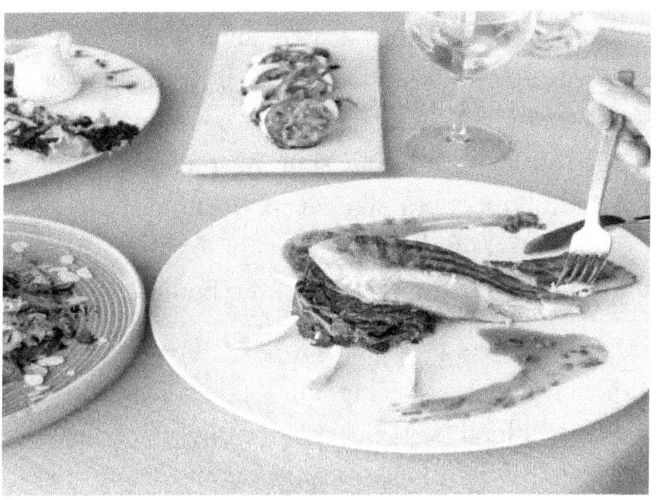

Be Mindful of What You Put Into Your Body

Blindly following fad diets, starving yourself, or grabbing quick convenience meals can make your body feel terrible. Over time, you can become desensitized to your body's cues that let you know something isn't great for you. Being mindful of what you put in and on your body will allow you to connect with what your body truly needs rather than trying to keep yourself fed or aesthetically pleasing to others.

Take time to notice how certain scents make you feel queasy or give you a minor headache; feel how your body changes as you put sugar into it; and ask yourself what your body truly needs when you are hungry or craving something. Your body has different needs throughout your cycle, and you need to be mindful of them each day and week. By being conscious of your body, you can learn to nourish all areas of it properly.

Allow your Body to Breathe

We spend so much time physically and metaphorically covering ourselves up that we often don't allow our bodies to breathe. The air we breathe and feel against our skin is healing and nourishing; in some sense, our skin must also be allowed to breathe. Mindful practices like deep breathing exercises flood our lungs and bloodstream with oxygen as we consciously exhale carbon dioxide out of our bodies.

Sitting in a breeze lets us connect with nature and explore new sensations. Likewise, freeing our bodies of restrictive clothing promotes blood supply, skin healing, and surface nerve repair. Sleeping with loose-fitting pajamas from time to time will allow your vulva area to breathe; this can also help prevent yeast overgrowth and promote good genital health.

Meditate and Move

Meditation is one of the most effective ways to control stress and connect with your thoughts and beliefs. Many women take time to pray throughout the day, and prayer is a form of meditation. Meditating allows you to become still in the presence of your own body, mind, and soul. With an examination of conscience, proper intention, and honest concentration, you can learn to love and accept your body with its shortcomings while eliminating self-limiting beliefs.

Movement and exercise are also essential for getting in touch with your body and understanding your needs. When you wake up each morning, try to do some light stretching or rhythmic movement while waiting for your morning coffee or tea to brew. To start my day, I like to spend a few moments in meditative prayer, do some light stretching, and do a simple strengthening exercise. Then, I head to the kitchen for coffee!

The Benefits of Working and Living With Your Hormones

Your hormones directly affect the quality of your life and profoundly affect your overall well-being. When your hormones are not balanced correctly, neither are you. While many of us may visit a doctor to check what is happening, others may assume that changes are normal and carry on with our lives. Neither of these responses may be correct. It's important to discuss your hormones with your physician, but we don't want to assume that we need to have a doctor prescribe us some medication to rebalance our hormones when we have a wide variety of options and solutions available to us that we can explore before we start taking artificial hormones or medication.

For women, each cycle phase is predefined by a specific set of hormonal changes that can change how we behave and feel at different times. Knowing where you are in your cycle and making minor changes to your lifestyle can directly affect your mental and physical health and allow you to tap into your hormonal superpowers. Living by your hormones comes with a considerable number of benefits, in addition to becoming physically and mentally fit.

A study conducted in 2016 showed just how important cycle syncing and living by our hormones is when a selection of women was assessed based on their mental and physical health over a period of time. These women, aged 25 to 46, were asked to nourish their bodies and exercise and work in accordance with their cycle. The benefits of the three-month study were recorded, and almost every woman in the study showed:

- a reduction in PMS symptoms.

- improved sleep quality.

- improved libido.

- increased fertility.

- weight loss for those who were battling to lose weight.

Additional tests showed that hormone balance improved, and the respondents reported being more energetic and productive and suffered fewer aches, pains, and injuries (Klebanoff & Keyser, 2016).

It's necessary to understand that people can't always be switched on and perform at their optimum. But because men work within a system that is designed for them, recovery is often a lot shorter for them than it is for women. When we can acknowledge that we have certain phases every month in which we are less likely to concentrate fully, feel less confident, or even do better with more introspective tasks, we can fully tap into our hormonal superpowers.

Your Period is Your Superpower

As you now know, your cycle consists of four phases within your cycle. In essence, though, you have two very distinct phases within your menstrual cycle, as determined by ovulation. The first is the pre-ovulatory phase, which consists of your menstruation, the post-menstrual follicular phase, and the ovulatory phase. The second is the post-ovulatory phase, which consists of the luteal phase. Your luteal phase is usually 11-16 days long, and you experience its early and later stages as you prepare for your ensuing menstruation.

Each of these phases involves changes to your body and brain. As you learn to live according to your cycle and become familiar with your body and the changes that occur within it every month, you can manage your symptoms, tap into your superpowers, and achieve your full potential.

Almost everything in nature is cyclical. The earth goes through seasons; trees will flower and bear fruit, waves will crash to the shore within high and low tide cycles, and the moon waxes and wanes from bright and full to complete darkness. Our cycle is similar, and accepting our natural cycle as we accept that the seasons will be warmer or cooler at different times of the year or that the sun will rise and set at various times every day shows us that we are made in harmony with our world.

To this point, I have explained the science behind your hormones and the shifts within each of your four phases, and you know exactly how each of these hormones affects your ability to socialize, how confident you feel, how creative you are, and how much energy you naturally have. In the previous chapters, I outlined what you need to do to remain healthy and balanced during your cycle and what tasks you should assign to yourself from a business perspective. In this upcoming section, I would encourage you to see what aspects of your personal life you can align to your cycle so that you are working with yourself in a personal capacity.

Menstrual Phase

Your active bleeding days may feel like the worst days within your cycle, but they also bring with them self-acceptance and an intuitive calm. It is perfectly normal to focus inward and have some alone time during your period to reflect upon what your intuition is telling you. While you are menstruating, it's a good idea to meditate upon your personal goals, visualize, and set your intentions for the coming month. Now is the time for reflective journaling, art therapy exercise, stretching, and meditation to discern precisely what you want to achieve as short-term, mid-term, and long-term goals.

Follicular Phase

Once your active bleeding has stopped, your estrogen will begin to rise at some point, and you may feel the need to clean your house or remove negativity from your life to allow for personal growth. Your powers of cognitive thought and your ability to concentrate and make decisions mean you may want to begin on some of your creative projects, spend time with friends who challenge you intellectually, or even declutter that room you've been avoiding. You may want to connect with your children creatively, teach them some life lessons, or bond with them in the kitchen while cooking and cleaning together.

Ovulatory Phase

Testosterone and estrogen are at their highest during ovulation; you're filled with confidence and vitality. With your self-esteem soaring, now is the time to go out and be social, look for a life partner, or hit the local karaoke club. If one of your goals is to get involved in a new exercise routine or join a sports club, this is the best time to do it, as you will benefit from additional strength and have the capacity to make new friends as your powers of persuasion are at their highest. At home, try new recipes, put on your favorite playlist, dance in your kitchen, choose color palettes for DIY projects, or get into your garden and spend some time reconnecting with nature.

Luteal Phase

Your luteal phase will have two distinct stages: one in which your energy levels are still relatively high and another where you feel your energy levels decrease as your period approaches (my.clevelandclinic.org, 2023). Large quantities of progesterone in your bloodstream during the early stage encourage creativity, and you can concentrate for long periods of time. If you want to learn a new skill like coding, writing, or studying another subject, your luteal phase is a great time to soak up all that knowledge. As you get closer to your period, tying up loose ends and decluttering your personal space will help you settle in and take time to introspect during your next menstrual phase.

Using your hormones as a superpower is so much more than being productive at work — it involves loving yourself, being fruitful and self-attentive, and living within your personal capacities. Living our lives through a male construct can be exhausting, and our hormones become unbalanced. We need to acknowledge that our bodies are unique and different from our male counterparts and that we have enormous internal power when we recognize and accept this hormonal greatness.

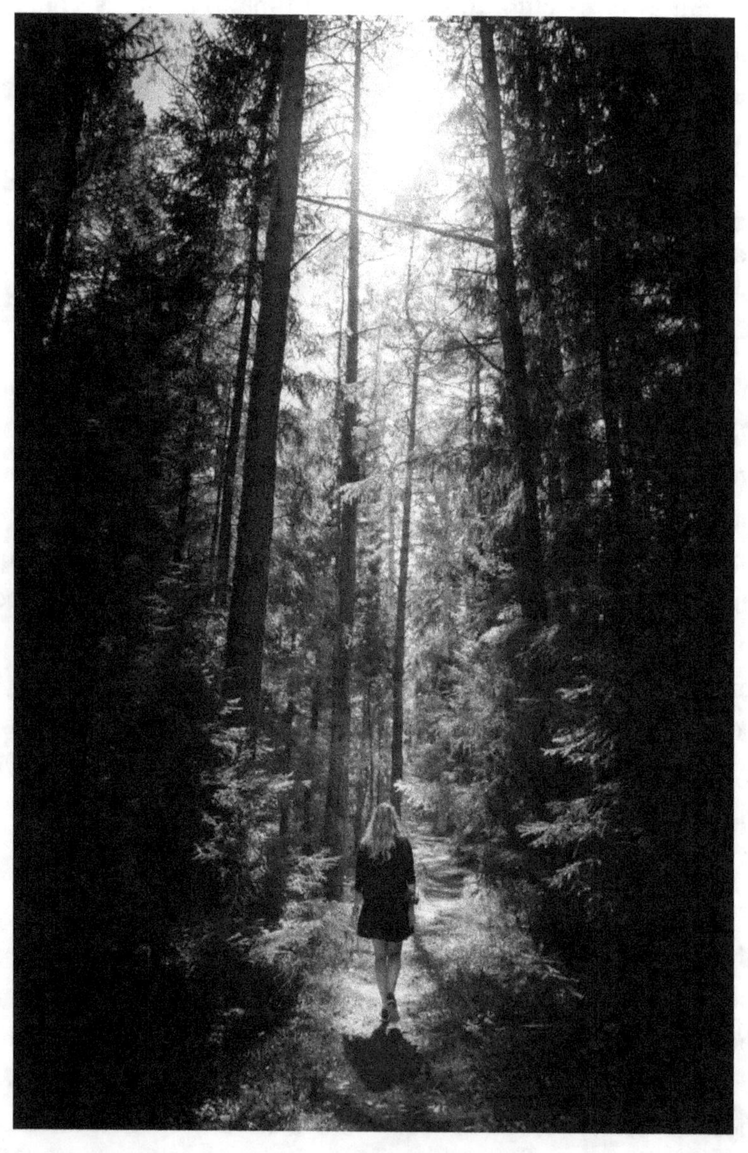

Chapter 7

Caring for Your Hormones Naturally

As our hormones are chemical messengers that affect our mental and physical health, it is important that we care for them in the same way that we care for our bodies and our minds. Your hormones always ensure you grow properly, your metabolism works the way it should, you are fertile, and your mood remains stable.

Under ideal circumstances, your body will produce the right amount of hormones and balance each one so that it works optimally. However, we don't live in a perfect world, and stress, a modern diet, and certain health disorders can all disrupt our hormones. In addition, as we grow older, some of our hormones will fluctuate and diminish due to the natural aging processes and other bodily changes.

Your body will give you signs and symptoms if your hormones are out of balance. Each of these hormones will be tied to a specific gland or organ. Some of the indications that your hormones are out of sync include:

- weight loss or gain that is inexplicable.

- muscle fatigue and weakness.

- general fatigue and weakness.

- muscle stiffness, aches, and pains.

- Arrhythmia, which includes a heartbeat that is too high or too low.

- increased sensitivity to heat and cold.

- excess sweating.

- frequent or infrequent urination.

- increased thirst that may or may not be associated with diabetic symptoms.

- insatiable appetite.

- decrease in libido.

- anxiety and depression.

- dizzy spells that include blurred vision.

- dry patches of skin.

- water retention in hands, face, and feet.

If you have one or more of these symptoms, it doesn't mean you have a hormonal imbalance. It may, however, mean that you should pay attention to your body and tweak your diet and lifestyle to see how it responds.

Should you be experiencing any of the above symptoms along with heavy periods, skin problems like dryness or acne, patches of dark skin called melasma, a dry vagina, painful sex, or chronic headaches, you may need to discuss them with your doctor or health care practitioner to receive a proper diagnosis of your hormones.

Hormones In Balance and Imbalanced

Hormonal imbalances occur for several reasons, and sometimes, the reason has to do with the hormone or the part of the body from where the hormone is produced or secreted. Some more severe cases of hormonal imbalances stem from eating disorders, trauma or injury, certain medications, being on hormone therapy or a hormonal contraceptive, diabetes, and treatments for cancer. Other causes can include chronic diseases like Cushing syndrome, Addison's disease, hypothyroidism, PCOS, and thyroiditis.

The percentage of women who experience hormone imbalances as a result of chronic disease is relatively low, and these women are usually aware of the issues they are coping with because the symptoms of their condition cause them to seek out professional medical assistance. However, many women who use hormonal contraceptives feel an enormous pressure to conform to society's beauty standards and are chronically stressed, meaning that a significant percentage of women may be experiencing hormonal imbalances that are imperceptible to them. Hence, they remain completely unaware of what is happening to their bodies.

Severe causes of hormonal imbalances should, of course, be treated by a medical professional, but women who are grappling with hormonal conditions can support good hormonal balance naturally, as well.

Balancing Your Hormones Naturally

Small, simple lifestyle changes can go a long way in rebalancing hormone levels for most women. Some of these lifestyle challenges were reviewed in my earlier chapters, but for you to truly support your body and learn to nurture it properly, we will discuss the topic a little more thoroughly.

Creating a life in which your hormones are balanced and you are living in accordance with your body can be divided into three lifestyle categories, and each of these categories will include some small steps you can take every day toward good hormonal health. Be sure to refer back to Chapter 4: Living in Accordance With Your Hormones for suggested foods and exercises to help you during each phase of your cycle (chegg.com, 2023).

If you are on hormonal contraceptives and you would like to cycle-sync, you will need to stop taking them. Expect to experience some bleeding over the next few days as your body adjusts to their secession. If you are on HRT or taking medications that affect your cycle or hormone balances, and you would like to learn to live in accordance with your natural hormones, speak with your healthcare professional about making these changes. You can embark on a new journey of living in accordance with your hormones.

Diet

Your nutrition may be the most potent weapon against hormonal imbalances. Not only does diet help nourish your body properly, but it also supports your gut health and ensures your body is creating, synthesizing, and absorbing the right vitamins and minerals needed for optimal health. Aside from the foods you can eat to help support your cycle, as mentioned in Chapter 4, your diet should be as rich, varied, and balanced as possible.

And I get it; life can be frantic and stressful, so creating healthy, nutritious meals from scratch can be challenging. But you don't need to be a victim of your circumstances. Meal prepping is a great way to ensure you're not spending hours in the kitchen every day, and healthy meal delivery services are available in many places. Please be aware that 'healthy options' on fast food menus often contain ridiculous amounts of sugar and salt that can damage your overall health if eaten regularly.

Here is what you could aim for when it comes to properly nourishing your diet.

- Eat protein with every meal: I don't mean having a big piece of red meat every time you eat, but you do need to ensure you are eating enough protein daily. Your body cannot make its own peptide hormones, and it needs protein to help sustain your energy levels, balance your metabolism, help you manage stress, and ensure growth on a cellular level. Plenty of plant and animal proteins are available to you that can be easily incorporated into your meals, like chickpeas, some nuts, and even peanut butter.

- Eat cruciferous vegetables daily: They are high in the phytochemical Indole-3-carbinol, which is essential for liver support and clearing out spent hormones in the body.

- Eat fruit but lower your sugar intake: Not all sugar is created equal, and while fruits do contain sugar, it's not the same as consuming processed sugar. Eating fruits with their skins feeds your gut microbiome with prebiotic foods and keeps your sugar levels in check. Be sure to clean them. Some people use a spray cleaner specifically designed to remove chemicals and wax from fruit skins.

- Some dried fruits like raisins and apricots: These are excellent plant iron sources, but make sure they are not coated in sugar. Processed sugars should be avoided as much as possible as they cause sugar spikes and imbalances in gut microbiota.

- Eat healthy fats daily to maintain hormone balance: Fats in foods are not something to fear, nor do they make you put on weight. Eating a good balance of healthy plant and animal-based fats ensures your body can fight inflammation and balance out hormones.

- Healthy fats include nuts, seeds, and avocados: Consume healthy oils like coconut and cold-pressed olive oil, sunflower seeds, and nuts (heartfoundation.org, 2023). Animal fats are not necessarily bad either, and certain fish, eggs, and whole dairy can do wonders for your body.

- Eat your fiber: Fiber can significantly regulate and maintain your gut health, ensuring your body can regulate insulin. Foods like lentils, legumes, and beans are all great sources of fiber and phytoestrogens that mimic your body's natural estradiol hormones.

- Be mindful of your gut microbiota: Gut health has a massive role in your physical and mental well-being. Taking care of your gut includes eating prebiotic and probiotic foods. Aim to eat various colorful vegetables throughout your week to help your gut bacteria thrive and maintain their healthy balance.

- Keep an eye on your weight: While I am not an advocate for unhealthy body standards, it is important that you keep your weight in check. A common misconception about weight is that an unhealthy weight means you are overweight. The reality is that you can be really thin and still have a dangerously high body fat percentage or that you can have too little body fat, which is dangerous for your body (inbodyusa.com, 2023). Being mindful of your body and understanding that your weight does not reflect your body fat percentage will help you keep your hormones in balance.

Exercise

Women have been conditioned to turn to artificial supplements and medications to try to balance their hormones, reduce stress, and be as productive as possible. But the whey protein shakes you're drinking to help increase your protein intake may actually have less protein than one and a half servings of Greek yogurt.

The reality is that the nutritional supplement industry is a multi-billion-dollar money-making machine, and just about everything available in the supplements you are taking is also available in raw foods. Most dietary supplements rely on the "convenience" aspect, but it can take less time to open your tub of Greek yogurt than it does to measure your protein shake scoops.

When exercising, it is vitally important to fuel your body properly so that you can treat hormone-related health issues and restore a healthy balance. Exercise has been shown to help improve sleep and with stress, depression, and mood swings, which are often the cause of and are caused by hormonal imbalances.

Exercise causes your body to produce more hormones. These include dopamine, which decreases stress and depression and makes you feel good; serotonin, which aids in good-quality sleep; and estrogen, which helps keep cholesterol levels in check and improves heart health.

The human body is designed to function optimally, and dynamic exercise, where we engage in some movement each day, keeps our hormones balanced. When you exercise in accordance with your cycle, you will incorporate different exercises into your lifestyle during each cycle phase, which will facilitate proper hormone balance.

In addition, you should incorporate different forms of cardiovascular and resistance training and preferably stretch daily. High-intensity exercise, while having many benefits and is very popular at the moment, can be detrimental to the female body during some phases, especially as women get older and estrogen levels begin to decrease. However, you can modify your exercise to include some high-intensity exercise. Swimming laps at a leisurely pace and incorporating swimming sprints, for example, is a fantastic form of high-intensity training that doesn't strain your joints. Gentle resistance exercises like Pilates are also easy on your joints but continue to ensure you get all the strength and mobility training you need to work your muscles properly while still balancing your hormones.

When it comes to exercise, consistency is crucial to maintaining balanced hormones, but you don't need to go all out every time you exercise. Instead, sync your exercise routine with your cycle, and if you're someone who doesn't use a gym, look for at-home activities that will get you moving. Gardening with enthusiasm, doing your housework to keep fit, and even just dancing in your living room are amazing ways to get some resistance and cardio training done on a daily basis. And remember to stretch, for even in the comfort of your own home, it will complete your daily workout. It really doesn't matter how you choose to exercise. If you get 150 minutes of moderate to intense exercise weekly, your hormones will begin to balance themselves out.

Herbs and Spices: Nature's Medicine

As women, we tend to experience more hormonal imbalances than our male counterparts, particularly as we try to fit within a male-centered work environment. Our bodies are designed to be sensitive to the hormones we produce, and if these hormones are imbalanced, we can experience some unpleasant side effects.

Years ago, before the advent of Western medicine, women turned to nature to help heal our bodies and balance our systems. Modern science agrees that certain herbs, foods, and spices profoundly affect our body's ability to balance out our hormones. By connecting to nature and using what it has provided to help rebalance our hormones, we can find natural, healthy ways to reduce negative hormonal symptoms and honor our bodies. While some of these beneficial tools that nature provides us with are in most of our pantries, others may need to be sourced from local herbal medicine stores.

When adding herbs and spices to your hormone routine, follow recommended dose guidelines, as nature's medicine can be potent. Everyday herbs and spices like garlic, paprika, sumac, turmeric, and ginger may not directly affect our hormones, but they are potent anti-inflammatories that help calm our body's stress and pain responses.

Flaxseeds are another great addition to your diet. Rich in antioxidants and phytoestrogens, these little seeds help balance hormones. The outer shell of flaxseeds is callous, so it's a good idea to put them through a grinder before consuming them or soak them to help digestion.

Maca is an adaptogen, which means it does not directly contain hormones but does contain elements that help support hormone production. This herb has been used for centuries to regulate and support thyroid function. It may help post-menopausal women with estrogen-deficient symptoms like night sweats and vaginal dryness.

Evening primrose oil, taken orally, has been used since its discovery to help treat health issues in the female body. Science suggests this is because the herb contains a host of healthy fatty acids supporting hormone function and reducing PMS symptoms. Evening primrose oil is also a powerful fertility enhancer that helps increase the production of cervical mucus, making the vagina and cervix a more friendly environment for sperm.

Shatavari is an herb used in Ayurvedic herbal medicine to help balance and support female hormones. This herb assists in the modulation of estrogen and improves PMS symptoms, as well as decreases blood loss in women who experience heavy periods.

Chaste berries and trees have also been used for centuries to improve ovarian health and naturally boost the production of progesterone, especially in women who are estrogen-dominant due to chronic diseases like PCOS.

Finally, motherwort and St. John's wort help regulate menstruation, reduce menstrual cramps, and treat PMS symptoms, such as disrupted sleep, low mood, and low energy levels.

While herbal medicine is fantastic for helping balance your hormones, you must understand that it can be incredibly powerful and may interact with and affect any modern medication you may be taking. Always consult with your healthcare professional before taking herbal medicine to ensure you are not canceling out or enhancing the effects of any chronic medication you have been prescribed.

Consuming some herbal remedies may result in unpleasant side effects, such as flaxseed causing loose bowel movements when taken in large quantities. So always be mindful of what you put into your body and be prepared to research your new naturals.

Everyday Foods That May Be Hurting Your Hormone Balance

To balance your hormones, you also need to be on the lookout for everyday products in your home that may be disrupting them. Trying to maintain hormone balance while still exposing your body to hormone disruptors is counterintuitive and will mean you're constantly attempting to correct an issue that you're imposing on yourself. But most of the time, we're unaware of these everyday items and what they do to our bodies.

For example, fruits and vegetables from the nightshade family may contain some great nutrients. But they also contain alkaloid chemicals that can cause terrible hormone disruptions and even death when consumed in high doses. You may have heard that you should never consume green potatoes, but you may never have been taught why (linkedin.com, 2023). The reason is that when this vegetable is green, it contains high levels of these alkaloid chemicals, rendering them toxic.

The foods listed under Nightshades are healthy in small doses, but we tend to overconsume them because most of these foods are already part of our daily diet.

Nightshade foods include:

- white potatoes

- eggplant

- peppers

- tomatoes and ketchup

- tobacco

- cape gooseberries

- goji berries

Of course, you don't need to eliminate all of these items from your daily diet, but it's a good idea to ensure you eat only one serving of these foods each day.

I probably don't need to tell you that refined sugars are not great for you (chriskresser.com, 2023). The spikes in insulin that non-natural sugars cause in your body can cause havoc internally and may even lead to much larger issues like insulin resistance. When the body is insulin resistant, it causes imbalances in estrogen, testosterone, and progesterone levels.

Factory-farmed and unregulated animal products can also cause problems with our hormones because industrial food production requires hormones to be used to speed up animal development. Several hormones are utilized in the production of meat, dairy, and eggs, and they are known to disrupt the human endocrine system.

Processed white flour containing high quantities of gluten and sugar also causes inflammation and stress, activating the adrenal glands and triggering an autoimmune response. When the human body endures this chronic inflammation, it can lead to a dramatic dysregulation of hypothalamic-pituitary hormones, decreasing the production of certain hormones.

Breathwork and Mindfulness to Reduce Stress

When we're subjected to chronic stress, our health suffers in so many ways: heart disease becomes worse, our ability to control our stress level diminishes, and our hormones become imbalanced. We don't need to be captive to our stress levels, though, and there are ways we can manage and even control our stress responses to help us get our hormones balanced and reclaim our overall health.

Diet and exercise are critical parts of stress reduction, but there are additional ways to help you manage your stress through breathwork and mindfulness. Many think of mindfulness, meditation, and breathwork as spiritual practices requiring concentration and self-discipline. But the reality is that everyone can practice mindfulness, meditation, and breathwork and reap natural benefits from them.

There are several ways to be mindful and meditate, including dancing, slow stretching, or even something as simple as going for a quiet walk in nature or preparing and eating your meals with intent and a new appreciation for the foods you consume.

Another common misconception about meditation, breathwork, and mindfulness is that you are supposed to clear your mind of all thoughts. However, acknowledging your thoughts without judgment and accepting them as transient can allow you to see them from a different perspective freely.

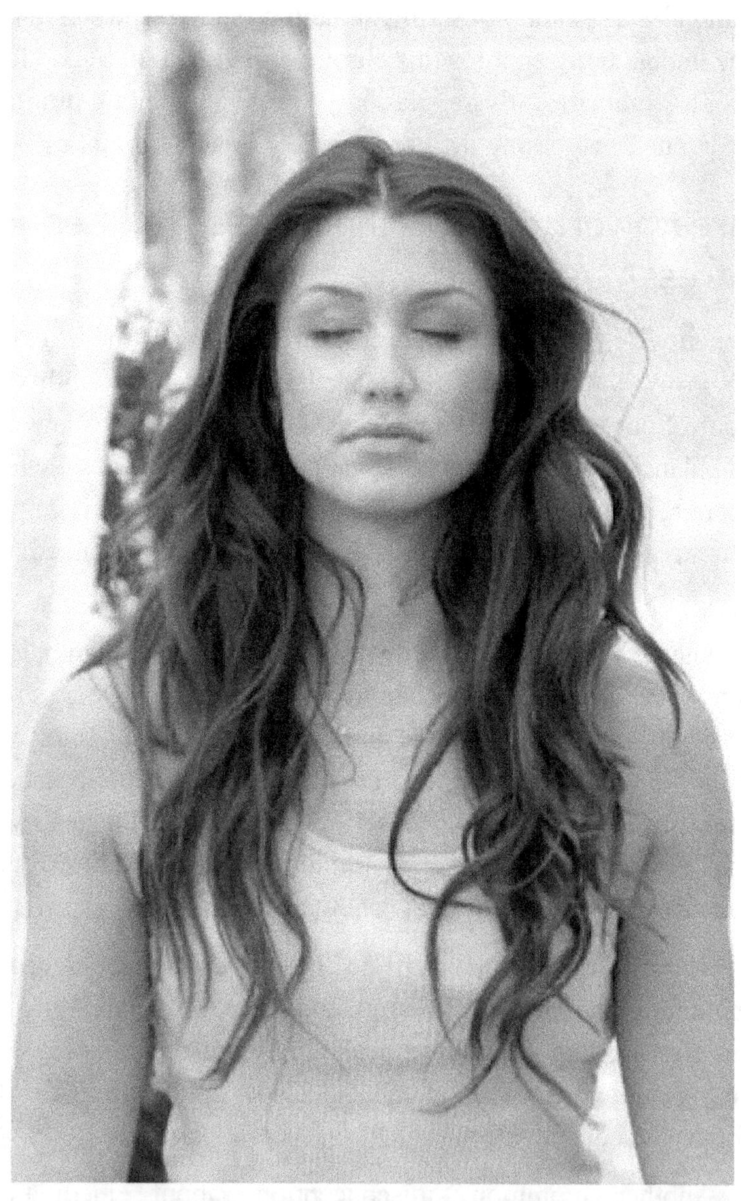

These practices help you reconnect with your mind and body, train your brain to accept life as it is, and can provide you with insight into structuring the life you want to create. When you can do this, calmness and peace can prevail as you recognize that your perceptions and self-limiting beliefs may have inhibited your ability to live in harmony with yourself (theguesthouseocala.com, 2023). Fear no longer compels you to control everything in your life.

The best way to incorporate these practices and work, eat, live, and exercise in accordance with your menstrual cycle is to understand that you are unique and that what works for you in your life may not function the same way for others. This means listening to your body and mind and making a conscious choice to acknowledge the value of your intuition in harmony with your natural systems and the life you were designed to live.

You can reclaim your natural state of being through a conscious connection to your mind and body, as well as the systems that keep you balanced and alive. One of the issues we face as women is that we believe we need to be all things to all people and tend to put ourselves and our needs last as we continue to try to take steps toward our own success.

We need to relearn that putting ourselves first to nurture our body and mind in the same way we nurture the needs of others is for the benefit of those around us as much as it is for ourselves. Considering our health needs and making them a priority is not selfish; it is essential because when we are the best version of ourselves, we can be the best version of ourselves for others, too. Indeed, putting forth the best version of ourselves often requires us to make great sacrifices toward those desires that inhibit our growth and interfere with our productivity. And I think this is the essence of true love.

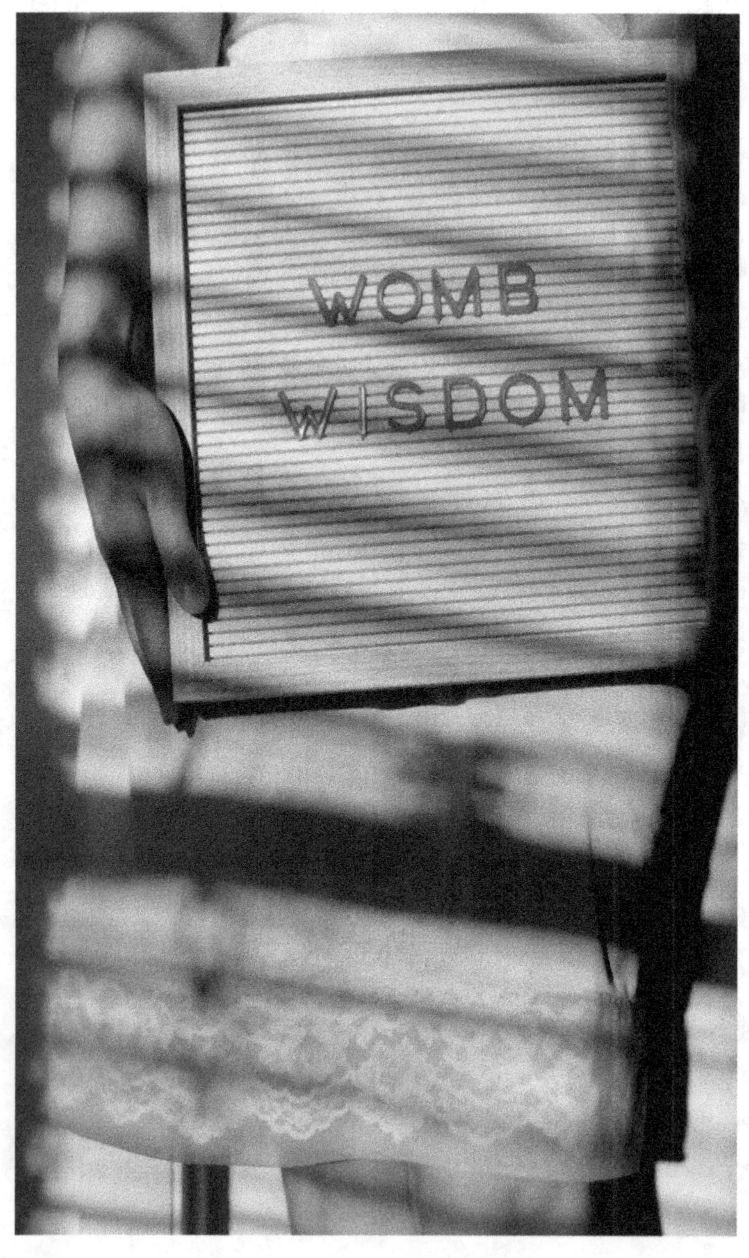
WOMB
WISDOM

Chapter 8

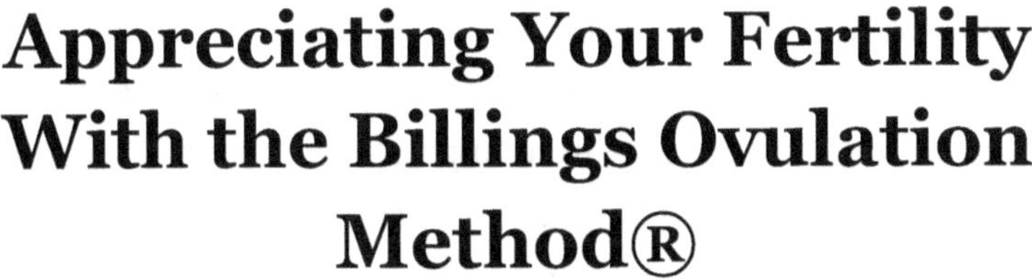

Appreciating Your Fertility With the Billings Ovulation Method®

Many women are aware that several fertility management systems are available to help us understand our menstrual cycles and manage our fertility naturally. These systems, often referred to as Fertility Awareness-Based Methods (FABM), are tools for achieving pregnancy or for postponing or avoiding it naturally. FABMs are resources that can empower us with knowledge about our bodies, helping us make informed decisions about our own health and fertility.

When we as women understand our menstrual cycle, our fertility, and what to expect from them, we are empowered to move within that knowledge to plan our lives, relationships, and families accordingly. My journey with FABMs begins and ends with the Billings Ovulation Method® of natural fertility regulation. As a young woman planning for marriage, I had the opportunity to learn this method, and its knowledge allowed me to gain a full appreciation for my fertility. I have used this knowledge to plan my family, space my children, and arrange my business affairs personally and professionally throughout my life.

I learned to teach the Billings Ovulation Method® of natural fertility management to many women locally and to help train women to become teachers of excellence, upskilling them over the decades as needed. And now, as an older woman entering menopause, I can honestly attest that its comprehensive application has afforded me a true and correct understanding of my fertility health throughout all the stages of my reproductive life, from my youth to progressing through my pregnancies and breastfeeding adventures and into my perimenopausal transition. Having aided hundreds of women in understanding their fertility, I am confident that you will find this method as accessible as I do, and I would encourage every woman to learn it.

One day, I hope to teach my youngest daughter the Billings Method™. She has Down Syndrome, but I think she will be able to learn how to monitor her menstrual cycle and record her observations, and I think it will be an excellent tool for safeguarding her fertility health.

I've been fortunate to attend several conferences, teacher-trainings, and seminars with Dr. John and Evelyn Billings. With each encounter, I have grown in my knowledge of fertility science and have shared this knowledge of the Billings Ovulation Method® with the women and couples I am blessed to teach. I greatly appreciate their work and dedication in developing this fertility management system and tirelessly sharing it with women everywhere.

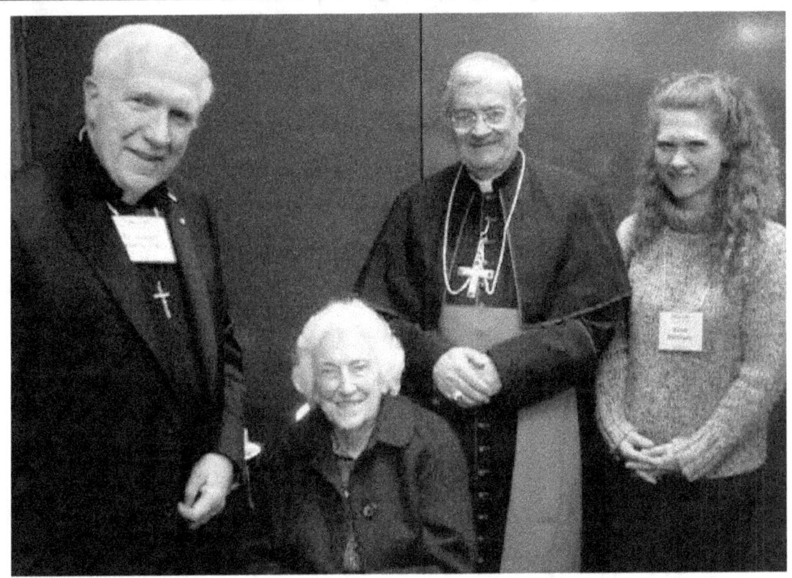

My hope for you is that you will see how this method of natural fertility management can help you live in harmony with your hormones and allow you to follow your fertility and infertility as you progress through your own menstrual cycle. Our menstruation is a beautiful compilation of structured sequences that progress a woman from a state of infertility to fertility and back to infertility in each cycle, as well as in our life's walk, working in tandem with our endocrine system and its production of our reproductive hormones throughout our bodies.

With the widespread availability of the Internet, WOOMB International Ltd. has made learning the Billings Ovulation Method® accessible to all women through their website. You can book an appointment to meet with an instructor in person or online, depending on where you are in the world. Women can search for an accredited teacher in their country and region or request to learn the Billings Method™ online. You can visit www.woombinternational.org or www.billings.life for more information.

Currently, WOOMB International has approved three digital applications to be used with the Billings Ovulation Method®. The Billings App and the NFP Charting Online App are designed to be downloaded onto a mobile device, while Fertility Pinpoint is a web-based program designed to be used from a desktop or laptop computer, or from a browser on your mobile device. You can visit your mobile App stores for the first two Apps and visit www.fertilitypinpoint.com to download the web-based program.

The History of Natural Fertility Regulation

The Billings Ovulation Method® is the first and oldest fertility awareness-based method because it was the first method to specifically use a woman's observations of her menstrual cycle to determine when she entered her days of fertility and when she left them. Before the Billings Ovulation Method® was developed, the natural methods of fertility regulation were known as natural family planning methods; these were the calendar-based menstrual cycle method, the Rhythm Method, and the Basal Body Temperature (BBT) Method (pubmed.ncbi.nlm.nih.gov, 2023).

Though sometimes effective, the Rhythm Method didn't work for many women, as it was based on the annual calendar with the assumption that ovulation regularly occurred on Day 14 of every woman's menstrual cycle. As abstinence was to occur during this fertile period of time, it was assumed that a woman wouldn't become pregnant if she refrained from sexual intercourse for seven days before and seven days after her Day 14. However, many unexpected pregnancies did occur, as ovulation doesn't always happen on Day 14 of the cycle for every woman.

To further complicate the calendar-based method's application, women do not necessarily ovulate on the same day in their cycle each month. Also, significant variations in cycle length and other factors like stress, lifestyle, and illness all meant that the Rhythm Method led to an extremely high rate of failure in postponing pregnancy.

When Dr John Billings first developed the Ovulation Method in 1953, it revolutionized natural fertility regulation. He recognized that the menstrual cycle has two main phases: the pre-ovulatory phase and the post-ovulatory phase (Brown, 2000). And he realized that a reliable biological marker for fertility had to be found (Billings, 2011). So, he focused on the previously known biomarker of copious cervical secretion to provide him with an identifiable indicator to conduct his research on women's fertility. Through the cooperation of many women, Dr. Billings established specific guidelines to help couples manage their fertility, which became the basis of the Ovulation Method. As this method evolved, the Rhythm Method fell out of use. While the Basal Body Temperature Method is currently still in use, its application provides postovulatory information, and it requires a rather stringent regime that is not very practical for most mothers to use.

In 1964, Dr. Billings published The Ovulation Method. From then on, he traveled the world with his wife, Dr. Evelyn Billings, teaching the Method to doctors, nurses, and women everywhere.

In 1976, the World Health Organization (W.H.O.) trialed

The Ovulation Method for three years in five distinct countries: New Zealand, India, Ireland, El Salvador, and The Philippines. The results were outstanding, indicating the effectiveness of the Method in the postponement of pregnancy as being 97.2% – 97.8% accurate. After the trial was completed in 1978 (Billings, 2011) and published in 1981, the W.H.O. recommended that the Drs. Billings attached their surname to the Ovulation Method to distinguish it from other natural methods of family planning, and its name was revised to the Billings Ovulation Method®.

According to studies published in 1995 and 1997 by the Indian Council of Medical Research Task Force on NFP and the Jiangsu Family Health Institute, China, the Method is deemed 99% effective in postponing pregnancy. Now, with more than 70 years of research, refinement, and hormonal studies supporting the Billings Ovulation Method®, it remains the most reliable form of postponing or avoiding pregnancy for sexually active couples. As Dr. Lyn Billings is known to have professed, this is "knowledge that every woman ought to have."

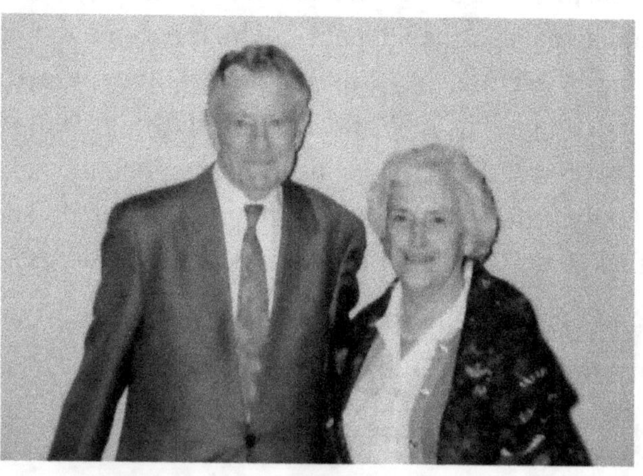

All modern fertility awareness-based methods rely on the early science developed through the Ovulation Method and the research that initially supported its development, including those that have been modeled on it. Currently, the Billings Ovulation Method® is used by millions of women in over 100 countries worldwide to assist them in achieving or postponing pregnancy naturally, according to their needs, wants, and desires.

A Simple Guide to the Billings Ovulation Method®

WOOMB International Ltd. (www.woombinternational.org) is an Australian nonprofit organization situated in Melbourne. It is the governing body of the Billings Ovulation Method® of natural fertility regulation worldwide. The Billings Ovulation Method® and its Rules are the intellectual property and material of WOOMB International Ltd. Their mission is to promote the authentic Billings Ovulation Method® in support of couples, the family, and society. They have recently published *A Simple Guide to the Billings Ovulation Method®* in 2023, and I would encourage you to find out more about it.

Learning the Billings Ovulation Method® is best accomplished with a qualified, accredited teacher who can assist you as you grow in confidence with an understanding of your fertility and the application of its four comprehensive Rules. Our Billings Method™ instructors provide ongoing mentorship and chart consultation until you have sufficiently acquired a sound and solid basis in the Billings Ovulation Method® and you are confident in your observations and interpretations of your fertility. You can find accredited instructors in your region through WOOMB International on their website's Global Reach page at https://woombinternational.org/global-outreach/ if you would like to learn more about your fertility with their assistance.

LH Explanation by Professor James Brown

[Report on an Article* from the Reproductive Biology Research Unit at the University of Saskatchewan

comment by
Professor-Emeritus James B. Brown M.Sc. Ph.D. D.Sc. F.R.A.C.O.G.

"A new model for ovarian follicular development during the human menstrual cycle", *Fertility Sterility,* July 6, 2003

Waves of anovulatory ovarian activity as described by the Saskatchewan study were documented by hormone assays and published in the scientific literature during the late 1950s and early 1960s. Their existence has been known to the Billings Ovulation Method for more than 40 years and rules have been developed to allow for it.

The woman observes patches of mucus associated with each wave of follicular activity and is taught to distinguish these patches from true ovulation, which is associated with a more definite increasing mucus pattern followed by the Peak symptom. This distinction is important because confusion between the two events could lead to mistakes in timing ovulation and this applies both to the avoidance and achievement of pregnancy.

Thus, the facts revealed in the Saskatchewan study are absolutely correct, we are grateful to the authors for reminding the world that the waves exist and we ask them to continue with their studies. There are more interesting phenomena to discover.

However, their interpretation that their findings indicate that fertile ovulations can occur more than once on different days during the menstrual cycle is grossly in error. From observing the millions of women using natural methods of family planning and from the daily study of approximately 10,000 ovarian cycles in a large spectrum of women we can state that once ovulation has occurred another ovulation cannot occur in the interval to the next menstrual bleed.

The Saskatchewan study confirmed this in that all the women released only one egg during the study cycle and the only two who appeared to ovulate more than once had abnormal (infertile) cycles. This is also our experience. The problem is to define the day of ovulation correctly and it should be stated that conception could not occur in such abnormal cycles and that they are an important cause of infertility.

The emphasis in the report on the assumed possibility that more than one fertile ovulation can occur on different days during a menstrual cycle reflects the unwarranted hostility of the authors, the Journal and the current official opinion to natural family planning. It also demonstrates that preconceived ideas obtained from assisted reproduction technology applied to infertile women are poor indicators of normal reproductive mechanisms compared with the study of normally fertile women using natural family planning."

https://drive.google.com/file/d/1YxAfk_49_TkNq4DCkdH PuQJQrPMEYRA2/view?usp=drivesdk

Reference: "The Continuum"]

Protecting Your Fertility Goals Naturally

Mindful monitoring of your body and your cervical secretion will lead you to notice changes in your sexual health (verywellhealth.com, 2024). Vaginal discharge and cervical secretion are normal occurrences. Understanding your patterns of fertility and infertility will provide you with confidence in what you may be experiencing as healthy or abnormal occurrences and provide you with early detection of any health issues.

Cervical secretion aids fertility, maintaining the pH of your vagina and ensuring it remains safe from harmful pathogens. Changes to your cervical secretion within a normal spectrum of sensations, colors, and odors are healthy, and you might produce secretions that look creamy white, tinted yellow, and clear or seem stringy throughout the course of your cycle.

During your cycle, you may experience days of spotting or unexpected bleeding because of breakthrough bleeding or withdrawal bleeding. Understanding why this bleeding is occurring will give you confidence in your state of health without fearing that a medical issue needs medical attention.

But dramatic changes to your vaginal discharge that involve an unusual odor or changes in the color of your cervical mucus different from what you consider normal may be an indication of other health problems. Itching, feeling feverish or flu-ish, pain when urinating, or vaginal burning may be an indication of a bacterial infection. Inexplicable bleeding should be investigated by your doctor as it may be a result of hormonal imbalance that needs correction. Strong-smelling vaginal discharge that is green, yellow, orange, frothy, or chunky, unexplained pain during intimacy or near the time of ovulation or in the pelvic area can be indications of an infection in the reproductive system.

Being aware of your cycle patterns ensures you are ahead of your sexual health and can identify fertility issues with your body so that you can receive early treatment, if necessary.

The Advantages of Natural Fertility Management

While the female reproductive system is certainly complex, it can tell us what is happening at every stage of our cycle. Once we become accustomed to our bodies and understand the cues they give us, we can begin to respond to them and act according to where we are in our natural cycles. There are several key advantages to understanding your fertility and using that knowledge.

These include:

- the ability to accurately pinpoint when you are fertile or possibly fertile and when you are infertile with confidence to mitigate your days of abstinence.

- the ability to manage your fertility naturally without needing to rely on any fertility apparatus or internal and external barrier methods and artificial or chemical contraceptives.

- a deeper understanding of your cycle so that you can eat, work, and exercise in accordance with your hormones instead of fighting against them.

- a great way to observe and record your cycle and its patterns, which can help you maximize your productivity and plan your days, weeks, and months accordingly.

- a safeguard for your reproductive health in which you can manage your fertility on your own terms and conditions.

Preserving the Gift of Fertility

In a world of modern pharmaceuticals and artificial fertility management, many women are looking for ways to prevent pregnancy or enhance their fertility without having to put unnatural substances into their bodies.

Over the last decade, there has been a very definite move back to more natural methods of treating our bodies and the symptoms that ail us, and our fertility is no exception. Natural fertility management methods ensure you can take control of your reproductive system with surprisingly accurate results when you apply their tools for avoiding pregnancy.

Additionally, there are no side effects or health risks when using the Billings Ovulation Method® (parenting.firstcry.com, 2024).

I've included this list of benefits because I feel it is important that you know some of them to help you understand why it would be a good idea for you to embark on this journey to live by your cycle and understand the natural signs and signals your body gives you related to your fertility health.

- Because natural methods rely on following your body's own natural indicators and processes, you never need to use harmful or risky medication to try to control your fertility. No fertility management drugs also mean there are no unpleasant symptoms like headaches, bloating, and mood swings.

- Learning natural methods empowers all women as they become confident in living in accord with their bodies. When a woman can learn to observe the natural patterns that occur within her cycle, she can plan and space her family as she desires, and she is empowered to become the best version of herself.

- Irregular cycles due to stress, coming off chemical contraception, or a host of other reasons can be reviewed and better understood by learning how they may have affected your cycle and observing your cervical secretion correctly with the cycle challenges you may be experiencing.

- Fertility awareness-based methods enable you to avoid pregnancy without hormonal contraceptive methods or their unpleasant side effects and those of non-hormonal contraceptives. As you record the onset of fertility in your cycle, you'll know when to abstain from genital contact and sexual activity. Conversely, hormonal contraceptives can have several unpleasant side effects, including headaches, nausea, mood swings, and irregular or absent periods. In contrast, non-hormonal contraceptives, like the copper IUD, are known to cause heavy, painful, and irregular periods (goodrx.com, 2023). All these side effects are avoided, and you can take absolute control over your fertility.

- These methods are non-invasive, meaning you are drug-free, harm-free, and risk-free. The use of certain contraceptives can be incredibly uncomfortable. In addition, it takes time for the effects of hormonal contraceptives to leave your system when you stop them or remove them from your body and for your body to readjust to its natural cycles again, prolonging the time it takes to regain natural cycling.

- They can be used throughout your whole reproductive life cycle. Because every woman is different and her cycle is her own, these methods allow women to manage their reproductive health through all stages of their reproductive cycle in their uniqueness, including navigating their cycles while breastfeeding.

- When observing the biomarkers and symptoms of your menstrual cycle, you can learn how your body changes and matures as your lifestyle changes and as you age. This allows you to prepare for maturing life events with greater ease and can help you navigate the changing symptoms associated with the perimenopausal transition and menopause itself.

- Natural methods are relatively easy to use once women understand their fertility science and follow simple, common-sense guidelines. Women only need to observe and record their body's observations daily by paying attention to the biomarkers of their cycle, so they'll know how to interpret them and respond to them accordingly.

- These methods provide recurring opportunities for couples to discuss their intimacy and future family planning desires by presenting them with ongoing invitations to reassess their family interests each month, and they observe their combined fertility initiatives together as partners on their journey of life.

- Aside from their fertility management uses, natural methods are also low-cost and affordable for couples without ongoing expenses while being environmentally sound and ethically acceptable to all cultures.

- Observing your fertility biomarker of cervical secretion throughout the cycle helps you confidently assess where you are in your cycle. With accurate, careful attention to your cervical secretion changes, you can navigate the patterns your body reveals to you and be confident in your ability to recognize your fertility or infertility each day.

- Safeguarding your reproductive health becomes second nature as you are always aware of changes in your cervical secretion. It becomes an incredibly reliable source of information regarding your reproductive system, so you can detect abnormal and unfamiliar patterns that may develop early on.

But the Billings Ovulation Method® is not only successful in preventing pregnancy (go.gale.com, 2023). It is also used by couples trying to conceive a child and maximizing their chances of becoming pregnant naturally by pinpointing their highly fertile days.

To Baby And Beyond, Choosing Your Destination

Please know that if you've recently stopped using hormonal contraception, it may take some time for your fertility to reveal itself and for your body to return to natural cycling. Be patient with yourself while your body readjusts to normalcy, as it may take several weeks or months before you can recognize consistent patterns of fertility and infertility. And if you are actively trying to conceive, allow yourself time and grace to be patient as your body heals itself from the synthetic steroids and returns to a normal state.

It is possible to increase your odds of achieving pregnancy. If you're trying to conceive, these natural methods will help you understand your body's natural preparations for ovulation and pregnancy through changes in your cervical secretions. As you record your cycle, you become keenly aware of when you are approaching ovulation each cycle, and you can use this knowledge to enhance your opportunities for conception, using the days of maximum fertility to your advantage.

Every woman can learn to use a natural system of fertility management, whether she is planning to conceive a child, avoid pregnancy, or easily monitor her reproductive health. Learning to be mindful of their patterns of fertility and infertility, couples trying to conceive can maximize their chances of becoming pregnant naturally by pinpointing their highly fertile days.

Alleviating Subfertility

Having a healthy reproductive system is sometimes impeded by physical or hormonal factors, which may decrease a woman's ability to become pregnant. A successful conception best occurs when all of the reproductive organs and cells are healthy and viable: the ovum and the sperm, the endometrium in the uterus, the cervical crypts in the cervix, clear and healthy fallopian tubes, and an ovulation that produces sufficient hormone levels. Pinpointing the most highly fertile days in the cycle by learning how to recognize your patterns of infertility and fertility can provide you with the best opportunity to conceive naturally.

But being in a good place emotionally is another helpful aspect to consider for couples who want to conceive, especially for those who may be having difficulty in conceiving, as stress can act as a deterrent to conception.

Many couples endure complex challenges in trying to conceive. A couple may have trouble in this regard for several reasons, and I recognize that some issues will need medical diagnosis and assistance. However, I want to emphasize that a loving and congenial relationship is vital to conceiving.

In 2008, the Australian Doctor published a How To Treat article entitled *Natural fertility regulation – The Billings Ovulation Method* in which two of the Directors of WOOMB International, Marian Corkill and Marie Marshell, reviewed the hormonal basis of the Billings Method™, its rules, and using the Billings Ovulation Method® to achieve pregnancy naturally. "The Billings Ovulation Method provides valuable information for the subfertile couple, as it allows the woman to identify the time of maximum fertility in each cycle. Women using the Billings Ovulation Method are taught to be aware of the sensation of the vulva and any visible discharge as they go about their daily activities."

Many couples who have difficulty conceiving find that they successfully achieve pregnancy once they have learned when the most fertile time in their cycle occurs. The Billings Ovulation Method® has a 78% pregnancy rate for all couples and even a 65% pregnancy rate for 'subfertile' couples (Billings 2011). Even though some women may experience minimal fertile cervical secretion, they may still be able to achieve pregnancy if they can recognize and make use of their most highly fertile days. Knowing your fertility will provide you with the best opportunity to achieve pregnancy naturally.

As you may be aware, some couples seemingly become pregnant from simply thinking about having a baby! But for others, it is more complicated. Lifestyles and habits may contribute to these conditions.

When a couple is suffering from subfertility, it can be helpful to consider factors that may be hindering the proper functioning of healthy sperm and adequate ovulation and address them, such as STIs, smoking, chronic fatigue, cannabis use, genital abnormalities, and genetic disorders. Among women, low body fat or obesity, high levels of physical or elite athletic training, residual contraceptive chemicals, and age are some contributing factors to be considered. Among men, occupations such as cooks or truck drivers, which raise the internal scrotum temperatures and result in low sperm production, mumps or other infections, or erectile dysfunction, can also be factors inhibiting successful fertilization. For some couples, these considerations may not affect their fertility at all, but for others, lifestyle changes and new habits may be all that is needed to help them conceive a baby.

World-renowned Dr. Pilar Vigil of Santiago, Chile, collaborator, and friend of the late Drs John and Lyn Billings, Professor Brown, and Dr. Erik Odeblad, is a consultant to the Board of Directors of WOOMB International. As a Professor of the Faculty of Biological Sciences of the Pontifical Catholic University of Chile, she has developed several protocols to assist women and couples afflicted with hormonal imbalances in achieving pregnancy and has significantly contributed to understanding ovulatory and endocrinological dysfunction. Dr. Mary Martin of Oklahoma City, Ob-Gyn, is one of her longtime colleagues who has studied several underlying causes of infertility to assist her patients. She has developed a protocol for dealing with infertility issues for her clients in the United States.

There are many natural indicators and biomarkers that a woman may use to pinpoint her most fertile days, which can be used to help her achieve pregnancy. While fertile cervical secretion is the most prominent and prevalent indicator of a woman's fertile days, other beneficial signals that she may experience are vulval swelling and swelling in the inguinal lymph node near the femoral artery in her thigh. These signals can be especially helpful for a woman who experiences minimal cervical secretion and challenges in conceiving, as they can alert her of her most fertile days, pinpointing her ovulation.

The highly fertile days are the days closest to your ovulation, as they reveal themselves in the conditions of cervical secretion. As a woman experiences fertile cervical secretion leaving her body, she will know she is very close to ovulating. A woman's most highly fertile time is when she notices that her cervical secretion has become very lubricative, giving her a slippery sensation at the vulva. She can learn to interpret the observations she makes of her cervical secretion correctly and use this time in her cycle to have intercourse to conceive a baby.

Sometimes, with the presence of cervical secretion abounding and present at the vulva, a woman may become concerned that her fertile days are coming to an end for this cycle. But when she remembers that her body is producing this fertile cervical secretion in anticipation of ovulation to nourish the sperm and facilitate their passage into the uterus, she will recognize that ovulation is yet to occur, as it usually occurs after her body ceases the production of this fertile secretion and that, 'the best is yet to come.'

Of course, intercourse during any days when a woman is experiencing changing cervical secretion is possibly fertile and can result in a pregnancy. However, the best chance of conceiving is when the woman notices cervical secretion, which provides her with a slippery sensation. This slippery sensation is a key component to informing her that ovulation is imminent. This ovulatory event is recognized and confirmed when she has begun her luteal phase. The woman remains highly fertile for a day or two following that observation.

The first three days of the luteal phase are considered fertile, as there is still fertile cervical secretion within the cervix, even though the mechanisms of infertility have returned, and the woman doesn't experience the secretion. With the ovum now released from the ovary, there is ample opportunity for it to be fertilized before it expires within its 24-hour lifespan.

Sperm Life and the Sex of Your Baby

The sex of a fertilized embryo is determined by the sperm that penetrates the ovum. Male sperm carry the Y chromosome, and female sperm carry the X chromosome. Interesting characteristics exist about each of them.

Male sperm travel through the uterus and fallopian tubes at a faster rate than female sperm. If male sperm are present in the cervix when a woman ovulates, they will be more likely to surround the ovum before female sperm reach it, increasing the likelihood that one of them will fertilize the ovum, producing a male embryo.

On the other hand, while female sperm travel through the uterus and fallopian tubes at a slower rate than their male counterparts, they can live longer than male sperm in fertile cervical secretion in the cervical crypts. This fact allows them to 'outlive' male sperm and remain viable to fertilize the ovum at ovulation, which may occur as many as five or six days later, more likely resulting in a female embryo.

So, intercourse that is limited to occurring on the first day of possible fertility as a woman experiences her fertile cervical secretion provides her with the best chance of conceiving a baby girl. And intercourse that is limited to occurring on a woman's final day of fertility, the third day of her luteal phase, would provide her with the best opportunity to conceive a baby boy.

Most women, couples, and families are not in situations where this information and experience are sought and needed, but there may be some instances where this fact can be very helpful. The following example is a true story of a couple who decided to use this information to complete their family.

One of our Billings Teachers, who was very familiar with her fertility and the Billings Ovulation Method®, used this information to plan their second son. She and her husband had three children when they learned the Billings Ovulation Method® of natural fertility regulation: a son and two daughters. After learning about the ability to time an act of intercourse that would favor the conception of a boy or a girl, they decided that they would like to try to conceive a little brother for their son. As they knew that limiting their act of intercourse to the final day of their fertility within each cycle may affect their ability to conceive right away, they decided to allow themselves one year of cycling to achieve their goal. With each cycle, they abstained from intercourse during her days of fertility while approaching ovulation and on the first two days of her luteal phase, which she knew were also fertile. Then, on the third fertile day of her luteal phase, they engaged in intercourse with the hope that a male sperm would attain and fertilize the egg. They repeated this process for many months as they remained committed to their plan of having another son. Finally, they conceived in the twelfth cycle, and nine months later, she gave birth to a beautiful baby boy!

Though this information has been known for decades, and there is no guarantee of the desired selection occurring 100% of the time, a comprehensive study has been done to test the validity of this information. The overall results and success of male and female babies born were quite impressive at 94.9% when the information that the Billings Ovulation Method® provided was accurately applied and executed. Published in 2011, the study, *Successful sex pre-selection using natural family planning,* was conducted by Sr. Leonie McSweeney in Nigeria. I have included the study in this chapter, with permission from the Pro-Family Life Association of Nigeria (P.L.A.N), and its link in my References.

If you would like to learn more about achieving the conception of a baby girl or baby boy, I invite you to contact a Billings Method™ fertility instructor from one of the links provided at the end of this book or contact me directly. Aiming to conceive a baby girl or a baby boy may take much longer than planning to become pregnant, and it often requires much patience. As I noted above, it is not 100% accurate, and you must be open to knowing that you may be gifted with a beautiful baby boy instead of a beautiful baby girl and vice versa. But God is the creator of all life, and he has provided us the ability to live in grace with these truths.

ORIGINAL RESEARCH ARTICLE

Successful Sex Pre-selection using Natural Family Planning

Léonie McSweeney

Pro-Family Life Association of Nigeria, National Hqrs., Eleta, Ibadan, Nigeria.

For correspondence: *Email:* Leomcswe@gmail.com Tel: 08037167664

Abstract

The objective of the study was to test the hypothesis that gender can be preselected by timing coitus in relation to ovulation, the marker of ovulation being the Peak symptom according to the Billings Method. A blind prospective study of 99 couples wishing to preselect the sex of their child was conducted in Nigeria, using the Post-Peak approach of Billings Method for males and Pre-Peak for females. Research co-ordinators examined the 'post-conception' form within four months of conception. This form recorded the timing of coitus prior to conception, and from this, the sex of child was predicted. 94 of the couples had a child of pre-selected sex showing a method success of 94.9%. 78 of 81 predicting a male were successful (96.3%) and 16 of the 18 predicting a female (88.9%). There was one user-failure, a couple who wanted a girl, timed coitus as for a boy, which they had. The study indicates that where comprehensive instruction is provided, the sex of a child can be preselected with a high degree of confidence by timing coitus, using the Post-Peak approach of Billings Method for males and Pre-Peak for females (*Afr J Reprod Health 2011; 15[1]: 79-84*).

Résumé

Présélection de sexe réussite à travers la planification familiale naturelle. L'étude avait pour objectif de vérifier l'hypothèse selon laquelle l'on peut présélectionner le sexe tout en calculant la date et l'heure du coït par rapport à l'ovulation, le marqueur de l'ovulation étant le symptôme du débit maximum selon la méthode de Billings. Une étude prospective à l'aveugle de 99 couples désireuses de présélectionner le sexe de leurs enfants a été menée au Nigéria à l'aide de l'approche du post débit du maximum de la méthode de Billings pour les hommes et d'avant débit du maximum pour les femelles. Les coordinateurs de recherche ont examiné la forme de la « post-conception » au cours de quatre mois de la conception. Cette forme a enregistré la date et l'heure du coït avant la conception et é partir de ceci on a prédit le sexe de l'enfant. 94 couples avaient des enfants dont le sexe a été sélectionné, ce qui montre un succès de méthode de 94,9%. 78 sur 81 qui ont prédit un mâle ont réussi (96,3%) et 16 sur 18 qui ont prédit une femelle ont réussi (88,9%). Il y a eu un cas raté : le couple qui désirait une fille, ont fait le calcul comme s'il désirait un garçon, ce qu'il a eu en conséquence. L'étude montre que là où il y a une instruction compréhensive, l'on peut présélectionner le sexe de l'enfant avec une grande confiance en calculant le jour et l'heure du coït, à l'aide de l'approche du post débit du maximum d'après la méthode de Billings pour les mâles et le pré débit du maximum pour les femelles (*Afr J Reprod Health 2011; 15[1]: 79-84*).

Keywords: Family Planning; HIV Control; Obstetrics; Sex-Preselection

Introduction

In countries where the "boy syndrome" exists and a male child is often sought at almost any cost, an imbalance of the sexes occurs, with a preponderance of females, as couples with only girls conceive as often as possible until a boy is achieved. Parents of all-female families tend to have many more children than they would have had otherwise. In a high proportion of cases, having no male child causes family disruption and promiscuity that may lead to HIV infection. In at least one area it is the commonest cause of requests for divorce. This information is given anecdotally as peer reviewed citations are not available.

Ovulation and the Peak Symptom: The Billings Method, with a Post-Peak approach to preselect males, is used as a basis for sex-preselection, by timing coitus in relation to ovulation, the marker of which is the **Peak Symptom** of Billings Method. The architectural structure of the sperm-conducting mucus changes day by day during the fertile phase of the menstrual cycle, under the influence of the ovarian hormones.[1,2,3] The Peak is the last day on which the presence of fertile-type mucus is observed, having a distinctive slippery sensation and the appearance of raw egg-white (though not always clear in appearance), universally recognisable by fertile women.[3,4,5] The cross cultural WHO study[6] showed that nearly all fertile women, in both developed and developing world, *could recognise the day of the Peak in the first month of observation after instruction*. This marker of ovulation is used to attempt sex selection. Ovulation takes place on only one 24-hour day in any cycle, either at the Peak or within the next 48 hours[7]. With twins, both ova are released within the same 24 hours. An unfertilised ovum dies within 12 hours[2]. As demonstrated in WHO and other studies[3,4,6], once they have been taught by trained instructors, women understand the significance of this mucus symptom and from it can tell when they are fertile and within 48 hours, the time of ovulation.[7,8] The Peak of the Mucus Sign is the last day of any slipperiness. It was given this name because it corresponds closely to *the peak levels of oestrogens in the blood just before ovulation.*[2]

Y-bearing sperms, necessary for the conception of male children, are more motile and shorter-lived than X-bearing sperms which lead to female children.[2,9] If intercourse is confined to the time of ovulation, the Y-bearing sperms arrive more quickly at the ovum and the resultant child is more likely be male. Intercourse confined to fertile days prior to ovulation is more likely to lead to conception of a female child.

To conceive a male child, coitus should be delayed until after the Peak so that the ovum will be either already waiting or released soon. The author had been teaching Billings Method in its general applications to over 7,000 couples over many years before the present study began, some of whom attempted sex-preselection by the Post-Peak approach for males. Anecdotally that application seemed to be correct. The author also noted that if coitus took place on the night of the Peak *(and was not repeated the next day),* it resulted in the conception of either a male or a female child. This was possibly because if the ovum arrived at the Peak, a male child would be conceived, but if not until 24 hours after the Peak, a female child. However it was found from anecdotal observations, that if coitus took place at the Peak **and was repeated the next day**, a male child was much more likely to be conceived.

A retrospective study had already been carried out in 13 States in Nigeria by the author, for different aspects of Billings Method, including sex-preselection using the Post-Peak approach for males. This was done by means of a widely circulated questionnaire which elicited 404 replies. The replies indicated over 97 percent success in sex-preselection, but though encouraging, this was considered to be no more than an approximation of the reality, as it was presumed that all the failures had not being reported. *A prospective study was considered important in order to rule out subjective bias.*

A blind prospective study was undertaken. Its objective was to find the true success rate and every possible failure. With the objective of finding every failure, the decision was made initially that if the sex of the child after delivery was not discovered (as could happen if the parents no longer lived in that State), it would be considered a possible failure. There was almost one such case, but eventually it was discovered to be an early abortion. Of the three couples who had a female child instead of the predicted male child, one was a late abortion. There was some doubt about the sex of the aborted child, but for the purpose of the study it was included among the failures.

The Ethics Committee of the Catholic Bishops' Conference of Nigeria formally approved of the protocol used in the research study based on the fact that the

ability to preselect the sex of a child promotes marital harmony.

Methods

In three densely populated cities there are centres teaching Billings Method.[10,11] Couples attend who are either experienced users wishing to train as instructors or are learning the method newly. During the course information on sex-preselection[12] was explained and any couples who were interested, were invited to take part in the study. Billings Method was taught comprehensively by qualified instructors with many years of experience. As explained later, those wishing to preselect should not attempt to do so until able to confidently recognise the Peak symptom. Because of their high motivation to succeed, this precaution was always observed.

For the purpose of the prospective trial, three forms were used as follows:

- **Form A** explained all that was expected of those wishing to partake in the study, assuring fully informed consent from those who would do so.
- **Form B**, the Post-conception form, was to be completed by the couple, to record all acts of sexual intercourse, the mucus symptom and in particular the Peak day, so that the timing of intercourse in the cycle of conception could be assessed in relation to the Peak. The act of coitus was routinely charted the following night on the couple's daily chart. *This form, together with the actual charts of three or four recent cycles including the days leading to conception, was to be received and assessed by the study co-ordinators as soon as possible after conception - within the first four months of pregnancy.* Couples were also to state on Form B the desired sex of their child.
- **Form C**, the Post-Delivery form, was to be sent by the couple to the study co-ordinators after delivery, stating the sex of the newly-born baby.

All who requested the above-mentioned three forms received them without any obligation to finally participate. The couple did not have to explain their motivation which could be for themselves or to help their friends at a later stage. *Being given the forms did not make them part of the study group.* The study population did not include those who did not respond.

Sample size determination

The number of participants was determined simply by those who brought the Form B as soon as possible after conception and fulfilled the five criteria given below. The study group was made up of all who fulfilled these criteria which included a good understanding of the nature of the study in which they were partaking. There was no pressure on them to continue with the study and nothing to gain apart from achieving a child of the sex they desired and being able to help others to do so.

FERTILITY BUSINESS

1. At least one spouse should be *able to read and write English* to facilitate accurate study of the forms, even though this excluded large numbers from the study.

2. The participating couple, both husband and wife, must complete and *return the post-conception form* to the study co-ordinators as soon as possible after the onset of pregnancy. Those presented after the delivery were automatically excluded from the study. Being a blind study this was essential but was the most restrictive element regarding the numbers in the final sample. Many couples living far away found it too difficult to return simply to report conception. Some would return after delivery to express their gratitude, but late arrivals could not be included in the study.

3. Irrespective of the sex of the child desired by the couple, the chart should show that *sexual intercourse had been restricted to days that could be recognised by the supervisors* as suggesting the conception of either a male or a female child according to the criteria outlined in the *Methods* section below.

4. The post delivery form had to be retrieved, unless an early abortion had occurred, so that the prediction of the sex of the child that had been made by the supervising team before delivery, could be confirmed or otherwise. Two cases ended in early abortion and were not included. There was one late abortion and it is included among the method failures. If the couple did not send Form C spontaneously, the co-ordinators went in search of it and retrieved it in all cases.

5. Ultra-Sound – At the time of this study, ultra-sound was not available in the areas involved. Nevertheless this procedure was explicitly out-ruled for study participants. Furthermore the prediction was to be made within four months of conception, before ultrasound would have done so.

No one who fulfilled these five criteria was excluded from the study. Ninety nine couples fulfilled these criteria and formed the study group. Details of their age and parity are shown in figures 1 and 2. The many who received the forms and did not respond were not part of the 'study population'.

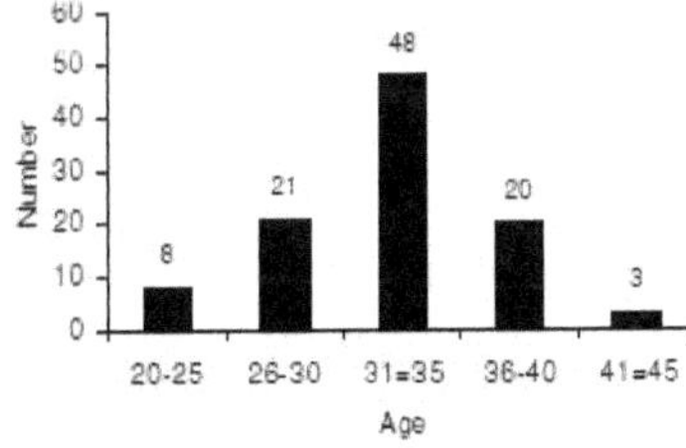

Figure 1: Age distribution of study participants

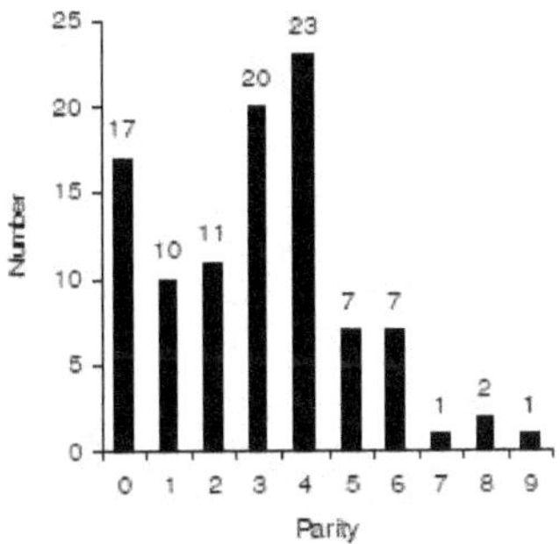

Figure 2: Parity of 99 women in the study group

The general teaching of Billings Method[12] was used to identify fertile and infertile days, using terminology suitable for use in Nigeria and a locally developed charting system. Participants in the study were advised to use only infertile days for sexual intercourse until they could easily recognise mucus with fertile characteristics and confidently understand the Peak. For this purpose it was recommended that they should avoid conception for at least three cycles. They were also advised to avoid conception until four months after weaning their last baby from breast-feeding, when a distinct mucus pattern would have returned. For the same reason, those who had been using the Pill or the Coil should delay conception until four months later.[13]

Confident recognition of the Peak is of paramount importance in sex-preselection. In Billings Method, **the** Peak is the last day of definite slipperiness whether there is any obvious stretching of mucus or not. *The mucus stretches much less at the Peak than on the days before it.*[3] The slippery sensation is caused by the presence at the vulva of fertile mucus, discovered by the simple observation of the slipperiness of *eggwhite mucus* against the outside of the vulva, during the normal toilet procedure following urination and without insertion of the finger. The vulva can readily appreciate the presence of this slippery mucus. Odeblad has demonstrated that "the sensation of slipperiness can be observed with 5mg or less of slippery mucus, which spreads over the vestibular area in a very thin layer, probably less than 0.1 mm. thick".[3] It is a striking sensation, easily noticed by busy women once they have been made aware of it and calls attention to its presence even when a woman is otherwise pre-occupied.

It is not possible to know it is the Peak on the actual day but only in retrospect. If there is no slipperiness the following day, the woman knows that yesterday was her Peak. The slippery sensation at the vulva is much more important than observing the stretching of the mucus. Understanding this is particularly important for sex-preselection. The Peak is the last day of any slipperiness. As stated above it was given this name by the scientists involved in the initial studies, as it corresponds to the peak levels of oestrogens in the blood.

The Three Zero Days: The three days that follow the Peak, when there can be dryness or sticky mucus (termed 'Pap' in Nigeria) but no trace of slipperiness, are referred to as the **Three Zero Days**. Conception is likely on the first day, less likely on the second Zero day and rare on the third Zero. Late infertile days begin on the morning of the fourth day after the Peak.

Rules used for Sex-Preselection: It is first necessary to ensure a good understanding of Billings Method. Illiterate women do not have a problem if well taught.

To conceive a female child: Sexual intercourse should take place before the Peak, preferably two days before the Peak and should then be avoided until the fourth day after the Peak. Once they have had some experience in the use of Billings Method, most women find that they can recognise the **approach** of the Peak by the changing quality of the fertile mucus.[12,13] Couples desiring to have a female child were therefore advised to begin their effort to conceive by using the first day of fertile mucus (*the first day of change from the dryness of the infertile days*), then in subsequent cycles bring the day of intercourse gradually closer to the Peak.

To conceive a male child:

- Avoid coitus *and any kind of genital contact* from the onset of possible fertility until the morning of the second day after the Peak. If conception did not occur, couples should proceed immediately to the next step without further delay, as conception is uncommon on that second zero day.

- The next step was to use the night of the first day after the Peak, that is the first Zero day, *and if possible*, repeat coitus the next morning. Couples were told to persist in trying in this way for about four cycles. If conception had not taken place by then, couples were advised to proceed to the last step.

- Lastly try the Peak itself, what was thought to be the Peak (knowing it is recognised with certainty only in retrospect) and repeat the act of intercourse on the following day. It was specially important to have sexual intercourse again the following day because coitus at the Peak alone leads to conception of both boys and girls.

The trial co-ordinators studied Form B within the first four months of pregnancy and on it recorded a *prediction of sex*, based on the timing of intercourse in relation to the Peak in the conception cycle. Later the desired sex recorded by users on Form B, together with the predicted sex, was compared with the actual sex which resulted (Form C) to assess the user success/failure.

Results

Method and User Success: Of the 99 couples in the study, 94 gave birth to a child of the predicted sex according to timing of intercourse, giving an overall method success rate of 94.9%. This includes the only User-Failure in the study.

Method Failures: Of the 99 participating couples, five did not have a child of the predicted sex, despite following the prescribed instructions. Three out of the 81 who carried out the instructions to have a male child, had female children instead. Two out of the 18 who timed intercourse to have a female child, had male children instead. These were the five method failures.

In one method failure to have a female child, coitus took place two days before the Peak and in the second case on both of the two days preceding the Peak.

Of the three method failures for male preselection, one resulted from sexual intercourse on first Zero day, that is the first night after the Peak, and the other two from intercourse on both first and second Zero days.

Method Successes: As stated above, the overall method success rate was 94.9%.

Male preselection: Of the 81 couples in whom a male child was predicted according to timing of intercourse, 78 gave birth to boys and only three to girls, giving a method success rate of 96.3% for the preselection of a male child.

Female preselection: Of the 18 couples in whom a female child was predicted 16 gave birth to girls and only two to boys, giving a method success rate of 88.9% for the preselection of a female child.

In this study there were no cases of twin pregnancies.

Timing of coitus for the 78 Method Successes for male child:

- 32 couples succeeded by using both the night of first Zero (the day after Peak) and the following morning. *Repeating intercourse the next morning, the second Zero day, possibly increased the chance of success.*
- 20 succeeded by using just the night of the first Zero.
- 4 succeeded by using the second Zero Day.
- The remaining 22 couples seeking a male child, succeeded by using what was expected to be the night of the Peak as well as the following day, the first Zero day.

The timing of coitus for both groups in relation to the Peak day and the number of successful preselections of sex are set out in Table 1. To determine the method's success/failure rate, the significance of the difference between results obtained with respect to the timing of intercourse and those that would be obtained with random timing, was assessed by means of a Chi-squared test. The CIA World Fact Book (Central Intelligence Agency of U.S.) gives Nigeria's sex ratio as 1.06 males to

FERTILITY BUSINESS

1 female. *Thus from 99 births, 49 or 50 correct predictions of sex would be expected by chance.* In fact there were 94 correct predictions. The discrepancy between predicted and observed values was highly significant ($\chi^2 = 78.23$, df=1; p < 0.001).

Table: Timing of intercourse in relation to peak in the 94 cases of successful sex preselection

Timing of Intercourse	Number of conceptions
FEMALE PRESELECTION	
Predicted Peak day minus 3	3
Predicted Peak day minus 2	6
Predicted Peak day minus 1	7
MALE PRESELECTION	
Day 2 post-peak	4
Day 1 post-peak	20
Days 1 and 2 post-peak	32
Peak day plus next day	22

Discussion

This blind prospective study shows that the post-peak approach of Billings Method is 96% successful in preselecting male children. It is more difficult to preselect a female child because of the uncertainty in predicting the Peak in advance; success rate was 89%.

Many of those who preselected a male child had either no male child or only one, until they began the "Post-Peak" approach. Of the 24 who had no male child before the study, four had two females, seven had three, nine had four, three had five and one had eight female children.

Studies compatible with present study

To the knowledge of the author the use of Billings Method with a Post-Peak approach for the selection of males, was first taught in the early-seventies in Papua New Guinea by Sr. Pauline Pitman. It was later taught in Nigeria in 1974 by the author. Neither knew of the work of the other until they met in Melbourne in 1978. By this time the nineteen women to whom Sr. Pitman had taught the Post-Peak approach for selecting males, had delivered 19 baby boys. Unfortunately this information can only be given anecdotally as Sr. Pitman has since died.

A study showing results at variance with this study was reported by Simcock[14], in which timing of ovulation was made by reference to basal body temperature which can only identify ovulation in retrospect[3], a likely reason for the failure to preselect.

Another study with results at variance was by Wilcox[15], the main difference being that coitus was not confined to a single occasion so that the act which led to conception could not be identified.

A special problem in the present study

As explained in the section on Methods, if conception did not result from coitus taking place after the Peak day, it is then performed at the Peak itself, but it must be repeated the next day, in case in that particular cycle ovulation was delayed till the following day.

However what was certain in this study is that for the 22 couples who had intercourse on what was expected to be the Peak as well as on the next day, a male child was conceived. *In contrast, of five cases who had coitus only on the Peak day, three had female infants and two had males.* These couples were excluded from the study as they did not comply with the study guidelines.

A big problem may arise for the husband in the last mentioned situation when many men are under tension and find themselves unable to repeat the sexual act the next day. The instructors were taught to carefully warn the couple of this possibility and how it can usually be overcome if they had previously practiced having intercourse on two consecutive days during infertile times, the wife helping her husband in this situation by what was taught as G, T and PPP, gentleness, tenderness, patience, privacy and play. [12]

There are two factors of major significance for sex-preselection that can easily be overlooked. The first is to recognise the Peak as the *last day of any sensation of slipperiness, even if there is very little stretching of the mucus, as the stretching is much less at the Peak than before it.*[3,12]

A second factor is that normal cervical mucus is crucial to the successful implementation of this method of sex-preselection. An important practical point is to ensure that at the onset of attempts to preselect, a normal mucus pattern has returned after breastfeeding, as was explained in the section on Methods.

The very high user success rate can be attributed to the high motivation to preselect successfully for legal, social, cultural and economic reasons. In some cultures parents of all-female families try to have children in quick succession in a desperate effort to have a male child before it is too late. As a result they have many more children than they would have had otherwise.

In these circumstances it seems reasonable to avail of natural sex-preselection to stabilise marriage, avoid a lot of unhappiness, have only the number of children they desire, raise the status of women, restore the balance of the sexes, and very importantly reduce the **danger of HIV infection** resulting from parents going outside marriage in the hope of getting a male child.

Acknowledgments

Particular thanks go to Drs. John and Lyn Billings for initial training of the author and later, while visiting nine States in Nigeria, for their advice to begin research as a blind prospective study. The author gives special acknowledgment and appreciation to Louise and Julian Ekwunife and to Paul and Helen Bobo, project coordinators, for their skill in teaching and their untiring efforts to help in the accurate acquisition, analysis and interpretation of the data required for the research. The coordinating team is particularly grateful to Dr. Bob Ryder (U.K.) for his valuable statistical contribution and his critical assessment.

References

1. Odeblad E. Physical properties of cervical mucus. mucus in health and disease. *Adv.Exp. Med. Biol.* 1977;89,216-25.
2. Odeblad E. The cervix, the vagina and fertility. *Billings Atlas of the Ovulation Method* 5th edition. Ovulation Method Research and Reference Centre of Australia. Victoria, 1989.
3. Brown JB. *Studies on Human Reproduction: Ovarian Activity and Fertility.* Ovulation Method Research and Reference Centre of Australia, Victoria, 2000.
4. Ryder B, Campbell H. Natural Family Planning in the 1990s. *Lancet* 1995; 346: 233-234.
5. Ryder RE. Natural Family Planning: Effective birth control supported by the Catholic Church: *British Medical Journal* 1993; 307: 723-726.
6. World Health Organisation. A prospective multicentre trial of the ovulation Method of natural family planning. The teaching phase. *Ferril. Steril.* 1981; 36: 152-158.
7. Depares J, Ryder RE, Walker SM, Scanlon MF, Norman CM. Ovarian ultrasonography highlights precision of symptoms of ovulation as markers of ovulation. *Br. Med. J.* 1986; 292: 1562
8. Odeblad E. University of Umea, Sweden. Paper delivered in October 2001 at The National Conference of the Ovulation Method Research and Reference Centre, Melbourne.
9. Shettles LB. Factors influencing sex ratios. *Int. Journal of Gynaecology & Obstetrics* 1970; 8: 643.
10. Billings JJ. *The Ovulation Method* 7th. Edition. Advocate Press: Melbourne, 1983.
11. Billings E.L., Billings J.J., and Caterinich M. *Billings Atlas of the Ovulation Method* 5th edition. Ovulation Method Research and Reference Centre of Australia. Victoria, 1989.
12. McSweeney L. *Love & Life: Natural Family Planning: Billings Method, 9th ed.* PLAN National Hqrs., Eleta, Ibadan, Nigeria 2002.
13. Odeblad E. *The discovery of different types of cervical mucus and the Billings Ovulation Method.* Ovulation Method Research and Reference Centre of Australia.
14. Simcock B.W. Sons & Daughters - A Sex-Preselection Study. *Med.J.Aust.* 1985; 142: 541.
15. Wilcox A.J., Weinberg CR, Baird DB. Timing of sexual intercourse in relation to ovulation: effects on the probability of conception, survival of the pregnancy, and sex of the baby. *New Engl.J.Med.* 1995; 333 (23); 1517-21.

Conclusion

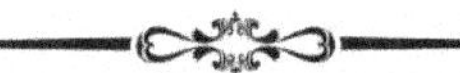

Over the last 30 years, while fine-tuning my skills in learning about my own body and the wonderful uniqueness of other women's bodies, my confidence and faith in the power of learning to listen to my natural cycles have grown. Understanding our bodies and aligning our goals with what our body wants to do naturally is extremely critical to our mental and physical health.

Whether these goals are fertility, productivity, and performance at work, learning to love ourselves, navigating perimenopause, or simply understanding how our bodies work so we can live life in accordance with our natural state, our hormones play an integral role in our ability to succeed at these goals.

Our bodies naturally wax and wane, much like the moon, as each phase of our menstrual cycle and our fertility comes and goes like the seasons. One of the issues we face as women is that we believe we need to be all things to all people, so much so that we put ourselves last with every step we take toward our own success. We need to relearn that putting ourselves first and wanting to nurture our body and mind in the same way we nurture the needs of others is good, right, healthy, and holy.

Taking care of yourself first is not selfish; it is essential in caring for others because when you are the best version of yourself for yourself, you can be the best version of yourself for others, too. More importantly, using nature and living in harmony with your natural cycle balances your hormones healthily and effectively without disrupting them with synthesized hormones that obstruct your cycle's natural rhythm and development.

One more consideration I would like to share with you surrounds the aspect of light sensitivity. Though we are strong and resilient in many ways, some women may be very sensitive to light, especially when trying to conceive a baby. And being light-sensitive at night could adversely affect our fertility, along with our sleep patterns. Mrs. Joy DeFelice, RN., B.S.N. P.H.N., has produced a study of clinical observations entitled *The Effects of Light on the Menstrual Cycle: Also Infertility* to this point. Though not scientifically peer-reviewed, the study has been discussed online by a few sources, and I've included the link to one source here: https://naturalwomanhood.org/light-elimination-therapy/

When we are sleeping, our pineal gland produces the hormone melatonin. While sleeping, light in a woman's bedroom can inhibit the pineal glands' ability to produce enough melatonin: light from a monitor screen or tablet, clock radio, charging port, or even streetlights or car headlights as they move along the street, etc. This lack of melatonin production due to this exposure to light can impact her hypothalamus and suppress the FSH in her pituitary gland, inhibiting its influence on the ovarian hormones of estrogen and progesterone.

Upon reading the study, a colleague of mine who usually slept in a darkened bedroom decided to do a little experiment with some light exposure in her room for three nights during her ovulatory phase to see if she would be affected by the change. She was not trying to conceive at this time. However, the unusual pain she experienced in her ovary was sufficient for her to recognize that she was light-sensitive, and she ended her experiment after the second night, not wishing to inflict further unnecessary pain upon herself.

Now that you have read this book and have plenty of new knowledge and information to help you live according to your hormones and intuitively take care of yourself, you can unlock your superpowers, too. It's time to elevate yourself by caring for your hormone health naturally instead of relegating it to last place and taking the steps necessary for your cycle's success.

By using cycle syncing, recording your cervical secretion, and using the tried-and-tested Billings Ovulation Method®, you can regain your personal power and effectively manage your fertility health initiatives.

There is a place for modern medicine, and you should consult with your healthcare provider if your body is showing signs that it is not well. But how would you know what those signs are if you're not fully in touch with your body and with yourself? If you want to learn the Billings Ovulation Method® for yourself and benefit from its time-tested treasures, contact a Billings Method™ Teacher in your area or visit www.woombinternational.org or www.billings.life to find one.

Taking care of our own fertility business is a necessary step in becoming the best version of ourselves and in caring for the people and the priorities in our lives. Thank you for making time for yourself and for making fertility business your business for life. And remember to nurture yourself to greatness, one day at a time.

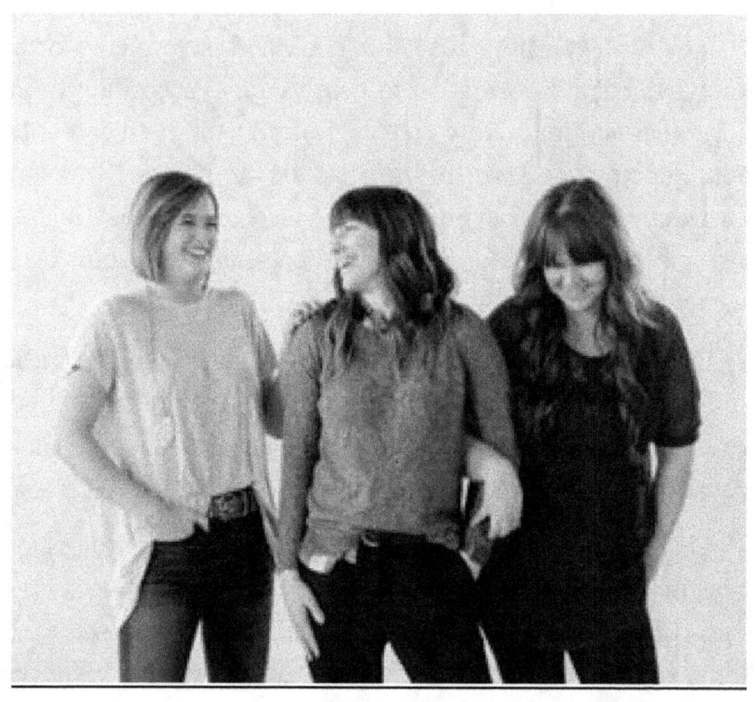

About the Author:

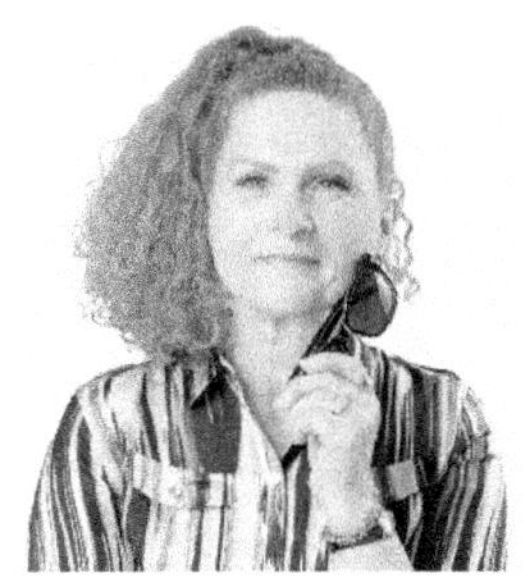

Anne C. Belanger is a Fertility Educator and Teacher-Trainer in the Billings Ovulation Method® of natural fertility management with the Natural Family Planning Association of Ontario, an affiliate of WOOMB Canada, the Canadian national affiliate of WOOMB International.

An accredited teacher with the Natural Family Planning Association of Ontario since 1995, she currently sits on its Board of Directors and is an active teaching member of BOMA-USA, the American affiliate of WOOMB International.

Anne served as the Administrative Representative of WOOMB International's NGO to the United Nations from 2016-2023, during which time she participated in several UN Commissions in New York City. The Permanent Observer Mission of the Holy See to the United Nations hosted her Presentation in 2017 and facilitated her discussions with international health ministers at the World Health Organization (W.H.O) during the World Health Assembly in Geneva, Switzerland, in 2019 (WHA72).

She is the Director of Fertility Business Initiatives Institute, a registered 501(c)3 nonprofit organization based in the U.S.

For comments or inquiries and to connect with the Author, Email Anne at Annatek, annatek@annatek.ca
Or annatek.com@gmail.com

Or visit

Fertility Business Initiatives Institute _The FBI of NFP

www.fertilitylife.org/contact

Links to a few Studies and Trials on the Billings Ovulation Method® of natural fertility regulation

W.H.O. A prospective multicentre trial of the ovulation method of natural family planning.1.the teaching phase https://www.fertstert.org/article/S0015-0282(16)45671-2/fulltext

Shao-Zhen QIAN China Shanghai Institute of Materia Medica https://drive.google.com/file/d/1k1L5SDZXzFeqYCxfdHK0w LRMFUDTtqv8/view?usp=drive_link

Indian Council of Medical Research Task Force on NFP https://www.sciencedirect.com/science/article/abs/pii/0010782 495002693

LINKS for Billings Ovulation Method® Teaching Centres:

Ovulation Method Reference &Research Center of Australia

(OMR&RCA) https://billings.life/en/

WOOMB International – https://woombinternational.org

WOOMB Canada https://www.woomb.ca

BOMA-USA https://www.boma-usa.org

WOOMB Mexico https://www.woombmexico.com/

Billings Method England www.billingsmethodengland.org.uk/

WOOMB New Zealand https://www.billingslife.org.nz/

WOOMB Egypt https://sjiforfamilyandlife.org/

WOOMBPHIL https://www.woombphilippines.org

The Billings Ovulation Method Association of Trinidad and Tobago https://www.billingstt.com/

Glossary

ADRENAL GLAND: This gland is located above each kidney and secretes the hormones adrenaline, epinephrine, androgens, glucocorticoids, and mineralocorticoids.

ADRENALINE: A hormone made in the adrenal Cardona, responsible for the temporary physiological changes that allow us to respond to stressors or danger.

ADRENOCORTICOTROPIN(ACTH): The hormone that stimulates the production of cortisol, which is responsible for our stress responses, the immune system, metabolic functions, and so on.

AMENORRHEA: The absence of a period for medical, age, or other reasons.

ANTIDIURETIC HORMONE (ADH): This hormone, made in the hypothalamus and stored in the pituitary, is responsible for constricting the blood vessels and regulating the amount of water and salt in the body.

ANTI-MULLERIAN HORMONE: The hormone produced by the female reproductive tissues and responsible for the creation of the testes as well as the ovarian egg reserves.

ANTIOXIDANT: Natural or man-made substances that can prevent or delay cellular damage.

BILLINGS OVULATION METHOD®: A natural form of family planning in which the cervical mucus is recorded in order to identify ovulation.

BODY SYSTEMS: A biological system within the body that comprises different organs that work together to perform specific life-giving functions.

CELL HORMONE RECEPTOR: A receptor for a hormone on or in a cell that is sensitive to that hormone. Cell hormone receptors are responsible for the signaling and receiving of specific hormones.

CERVICAL MUCUS: The fluid produced by the cervix which changes in consistency, volume, and texture throughout the course of the female reproductive cycle.

CORTISOL: The steroid hormone produced by the cortex's 'outer area' of the adrenal gland, which prepares the body for a fight-or-flight response.

CORPUS LUTEUM: A luteinized hormone-secreting group of cells comprising the remainder of the follicle after ovulation organized to produce progesterone for the support of an ensuing pregnancy.

CYCLE SYNCING: The practice of changing your lifestyle to match the four phases of the female menstrual cycle.

DOPAMINE: A hormone produced in the brain that is important in regulating mood and lactation.

DYSMENORRHEA: Abnormal pain associated with menstruation.

EMBRYO: The early developmental stages of a mammal within the uterus of its mother, up to 8 weeks post conception in humans.

ENDOCRINE SYSTEM: A system within the body that consists of glands and organs and which regulates and controls hormones. These hormones coordinate and control metabolism, reproduction, responses to stress, mood, energy levels, and so on.

ENDOMETRIUM: The lining of the uterus.

EPITHELIUM: The outer layer of cells that line hollow organs and glands and exist on the outer surface of the body.

ESTROGEN: A steroid hormone often associated with the female reproductive system. While biological females have higher estrogen levels, men also produce and use estrogen.

FETUS: The gestational time of a mammal, from 8 weeks until birth in humans.

FOLLICLE: A multicellular structure in the ovary within which an egg develops.

FOLLICLE STIMULATING HORMONE (FSH): A hormone produced by the pituitary gland that is essential for the proper functioning of the female and male reproductive system.

GLAND: An organ in the human body responsible for the secretion of natural chemicals and hormones.

GONADOTROPIN: A hormone that influences the pituitary gland to stimulate the production of the follicle-stimulating hormone and the luteinizing hormone.

GONAD: The primary reproductive organs of the ovaries in the female and the testes in the male reproductive system.

GUT-BRAIN AXIS: A two-way biochemical process that takes place between the central nervous system and the gastrointestinal tract.

HEART RATE VARIABILITY (HRV): The fluctuations in the amount of time between heartbeats.

HORMONE: A naturally occurring chemical circulated through the bloodstream that coordinates specific functions from the body's organs, muscles, and tissues.

HUMAN CHORIONIC GONADOTROPIN (hCG): The hormone produced by the early embryo and later by the placenta that helps to sustain early pregnancy until about 10 weeks of gestation.

HYPOTHALAMUS: A structure within the brain that controls bodily functions, primarily keeping the body in a state of homeostasis.

IMPLANTATION: The process by which the embryo attaches to the endometrial surface at the epithelium.

LUTEINIZING HORMONE (LH): the hormone made in the anterior pituitary gland that triggers ovulation.

MEDULLA OBLONGATA: The connection between the brainstem and the spinal cord.

MELATONIN: A hormone produced in the brain when light is not entering your eyes in response to darkness, which assists with the circadian rhythms

MENORRHEA: The flow of menstrual blood that is considered to be within normal parameters.

MENSTRUAL CYCLE: The female reproductive cycle.

MENTRUATION: The shedding of the uterine lining via the cervix and expelled out of the vagina. Menstruation occurs following ovulation and usually lasts three to nine days.

MITTELSCHMERZ: A benign preovulatory abdominal pain that occurs near the time of ovulation.

OOCYTE: An immature female reproductive cell.

ORGANS: Structures within a body that serve a specific function and purpose, such as the heart, liver, lungs, and so on.

OVARIES: A pair of glands in the female body that house eggs and produce as well as regulate the hormones estrogen and progesterone.

OVULATION: The phase in the female menstrual cycle in which an egg is released from one or both ovaries.

OVULATORY CYCLE: A well-ordered series of events encompassing the development of the follicle to the demise of the corpus luteum.

OVUM: A female reproductive cell developed in a follicle.

OXYTOCIN: A hormone that is made in the Hypothalamus but stored in your Pituitary gland and assists in the process of lactation, arousal, and attachment.

PINEAL GLAND: A small gland present in the brain that is responsible for the body's circadian rhythms through the secretion of melatonin.

PITUITARY GLAND: One of the major glands within the endocrine system that is responsible for the function of the body's other endocrine glands.

PREBIOTIC: Whole plant foods that serve as food for the microbiota living in the digestive system.

PREMENSTRUAL SYNDROME: The symptoms experienced before and during menstruation due to the premenstrual fall in progesterone levels.

PROBIOTIC: Foods and/or medications that contain beneficial microbiota for the digestive system.

PROGESTERONE: A steroid hormone primarily produced by the corpus luteum in women and the placenta to sustain a pregnancy, which is critical to reproductive health.

PROGESTIN: A synthetic progesterone-like drug.

PROLACTIN: A critical hormone produced by the pituitary gland, responsible for the production of milk in females and breast tissue development.

PROSTAGLANDIN: A natural hormone-like lipid created to mediate various processes, including inflammation and the onset of labor.

RELAXIN: A hormone produced by the ovaries, as well as the placenta, should a woman become pregnant. This hormone relaxes the muscles, joints, and ligaments.

SEROTONIN: A chemical messenger produced to communicate messages from nerve cells in the brain with other parts of your body.

SEXUALLY TRANSMITTED INFECTION (STI): A viral or bacterial infection acquired through unprotected sex with an infected person.

SOMATOTROPIN: AKA, Growth hormone responsible for tissue and cellular growth.

TESTOSTERONE: A primarily male sex hormone that is critical to the development and functions of biologically male individuals. Testosterone is also produced in lower quantities in women by the ovaries, skin, and fat cells.

THALAMUS: The gray matter in the brain that serves as the relay station for incoming and outgoing messages to and from the brain.

THYROTROPIN (TSH): AKA, Thyroid-stimulating hormone that serves to stimulate metabolism.

THYMUS: A gland in the upper chest responsible for producing lymphocytes that protect against bacterial and viral infections.

TESTES: The primary male sex glands, or gonads that are responsible for the production of testosterone and sperm and regulate other reproductive functions.

THYROID: The gland in the front of the neck that regulates the overall rate of bodily metabolism.

UTERUS: The hormone-responsive female sex organ that houses the growing fetus. The lining of the uterus sheds during menstruation if conception doesn't take place.

VAGUS NERVE: The main nerves belonging to the parasympathetic nervous system, which control numerous body functions, including heart rate, immunity, and digestion.

References

Ahmed, Z. (2022). Current Clinical Trials in Traumatic Brain Injury. *Brain Sciences,* *12*(5), 527. https://doi.org/10.3390/brainsci12050527

Billings, E., Westmore, A., (2011) *The Billings Method, Using the body's natural signal of fertility to achieve or avoid pregnancy* https://billings.ecwid.com/The-Billings-Method-by-Dr-Evelyn-Billings-&-Dr-Ann-Westmore-p36860362

BillingsLIFE. (2014). *The menstrual cycle and your body's natural signal of fertility - cervical mucus.* www.youtube.com. https://www.youtube.com/watch?v=0ldx6Nago6I&t=188s

BOMA-USA – Billings Ovulation Method Association. (n.d.). BOMA-USA. Retrieved April 17, 2023, from https://boma-usa.org/

Brown, J.B., Professor-Emeritus M.Sc. Ph.D., (2000) Studies on Human Reproduction: Ovarian Activity and Fertility and the Billings Ovulation Method https://billings.ecwid.com/Billings-Teacher-Resources-Downloads-c34707135

Davydov, D. M., Shapiro, D., Goldstein, I. B., & Chicz-DeMet, A. (2005). *Moods in Everyday Situations: Effects of Menstrual Cycle,* *Work,* *and* *Stress* *Hormones.* https://www.sciencedirect.com/science/article/abs/pii/S0022399904006439

Dyer, O. (2003). Women may ovulate two or three times a month. *BMJ : British Medical Journal, 327(7407),* 124. https://www.ncbi.nlm.nih.gov/pmc/articles/PMC1126506/#:~:text=The%20conventional%20belief%20that%20women

Foods to support your cycle in each phase. (2022, May 5). Nutra Organics. https://nutraorganics.com.au/blogs/blog/foods-to-support-your-cycle-in-each-phase#:~:text=Luteal%20Phase

Hashemian, F., Shafigh, F., & Roohi, E. (2016). Regulatory role of prolactin in paternal behavior in male parents: A narrative review *Journal of Postgraduate Medicine,* *62*(3), 182. https://journals.lww.com/jopm/abstract/2016/62030/regulatory_role_of_prolactin_in_paternal_behavior.9.aspx

Home - WOOMB International. (2021, July 12). WOOMB International. https://woombinternational.org/

Jennifer Knudtson. (2018). *Female Reproductive Endocrinology.* MSD Manual Professional Edition; MSD Manuals. https://www.msdmanuals.com/professional/gynecology-and-obstetrics/female-reproductive-endocrinology/female-reproductive-endocrinology

Kay, Dr. C. (2020, February 24). *What Is Cycle Syncing?* Healthline. https://www.healthline.com/health/womens-health/guide-to-cycle-syncing-how-to-start

Klebanoff, N. A., & Keyser, P. K. (2016). *Menstrual Synchronization: A Qualitative Study.* NCBI. https://pubmed.ncbi.nlm.nih.gov/8708350/

Mandalaneni, K., & Rayi, A. (2021). *Vagus Nerve Stimulator.* PubMed; StatPearls Publishing. https://www.ncbi.nlm.nih.gov/books/NBK562175/

McSweeney, L., (2011) *Successful Sex Pre-selection using Natural Family Planning* https://pubmed.ncbi.nlm.nih.gov/21987941/

Monda, V., Villano, I., Messina, A., Valenzano, A., Esposito, T., Moscatelli, F., Viggiano, A., Cibelli, G., Chieffi, S., Monda, M., & Messina, G. (2017). Exercise Modifies the Gut Microbiota with Positive Health Effects. *Oxidative Medicine and Cellular Longevity,* *2017*, 1–8. https://doi.org/10.1155/2017/3831972

Price, M. (n.d.). *Billings LIFE: Official Site of The Billings Ovulation Method[TM] - Leaders in Fertility Education.* Billings.life. Retrieved April 17, 2023, from https://billings.life/en/

Proctor, M., & Farquhar, C. (2006). Diagnosis and management of dysmenorrhoea. *BMJ : British Medical Journal, 332*(7550), 1134–1138. https://www.ncbi.nlm.nih.gov/pmc/articles/PMC1459624/

Roache, C. (2007, October 31). *Changes to Diet and Lifestyle May Help Prevent Infertility from Ovulatory Disorders.* Harvard School of Public Health. https://news.harvard.edu/gazette/story/2007/11/changes-in-diet-and-lifestyle-may-help-prevent-infertility/

Settler, Fred. R. (2013). Growth hormone in the aging male. *Best Practice & Research Clinical Endocrinology & Metabolism, 27*(4), 541–555. https://doi.org/10.1016/j.beem.2013.05.003

Silkin, L. (2021, July 6). *Women in Work: a brief history of women in the workplace — Future of Work Hub.* Futureofworkhub. https://www.futureofworkhub.info/comment/2021/7/6/women-in-work-a-brief-history-of-women-in-the-workplace#:~:text=The%20National%20Service%20Act%201941

Sims, S. T., Ware, L., & Capodilupo, E. R. (2021). Patterns of endogenous and exogenous ovarian hormone modulation on recovery metrics across the menstrual cycle. *BMJ Open Sport & Exercise Medicine, 7*(3), e001047. https://doi.org/10.1136/bmjsem-2021-001047

Straftis, A. A., & Gray, P. B. (2019). Sex, Energy, Well-Being and Low Testosterone: An Exploratory Survey of U.S. Men's Experiences on Prescription Testosterone. *International Journal of Environmental Research and Public Health, 16*(18). https://doi.org/10.3390/ijerph16183261

Toffoletto, S., Lanzenberger, R., Gingnell, M., Sundström-Poromaa, I., & Comasco, E. (2014). Emotional and cognitive functional imaging of estrogen and progesterone effects in the female human brain: A systematic review. *Psychoneuroendocrinology, 50,* 28–52. https://doi.org/10.1016/j.psyneuen.2014.07.025

van der Spoel, E., Roelfsema, F., & van Heemst, D. (2021). Relationships Between 24-hour LH and Testosterone Concentrations and With Other Pituitary Hormones in Healthy Older Men. *Journal of the Endocrine Society, 5*(9). https://doi.org/10.1210/jendso/bvab075

Watson, Dr. S. (2018, August 17). *Stages of Menstrual Cycle: Menstruation, Ovulation, Hormones, Mor.* Healthline. https://www.healthline.com/health/womens-health/stages-of-menstrual-cycle

Wharton, W., E. Gleason, C., Sandra, O., M. Carlsson, C., & Asthana, S. (2012). Neurobiological Underpinnings of the Estrogen - Mood Relationship. Current *Psychiatry Reviews, 8*(3), 247–256. https://doi.org/10.2174/157340012800792957

WOOMB International Directors, G. Barker, K.Bourke, M. Corkill, B. Davies, M. Marshall, (2017) Understanding Couple Fertility with the Billings Ovulation Method® https://billings.ecwid.com/PDF-eBook-Understanding-Couple-Fertility-with-the-Billings-Ovulation-Method%C2%AEDOWNLOAD-English-Spanish-and-Vietnamese-p97803443

Image References

Adam Winger. (2020). *Woman in gray crewneck* [Image]. https://unsplash.com/photos/oh6FswCTTmY

Ava Sol. (2022). *The way to maintain one's connection to the wild is to ask yourself what it is that you want. This is the sorting of the seed from the dirt* [Image]. https://unsplash.com/photos/UEhjwhoTmh8

Elisa Ventur. (2021). *A business woman who is stressed and frustrated* [Image]. https://unsplash.com/photos/I-uY25-Paj1

Ella Olsson. (2018). *Traveled to a remote village close to Lake Como in Italy.* [Image]. https://unsplash.com/photos/I-uYa5P-EgM

Farhad Ibrahimzade. (2020). *Cooked fish on white ceramic* [Image]. https://unsplash.com/photos/isHUj3N0194

Geran de Klerk. (2017). *Woman walking in the forest* [Image]. https://unsplash.com/photos/Kcxv7Gz7wmw

Kenny Eliason. (2021). *Editorial* [Image]. https://unsplash.com/photos/MEbT27ZrtdE

Lisa Yount. (2022). *Unknown* [Image]. https://unsplash.com/photos/JkAxfH5ktpw

Museums of History New South Wales. (2023). Working the industrial ironing machine Title: Industrial and Commercial Electrical Machines - Industrial Ironing Machine [Image]. https://unsplash.com/photos/nQBwIMHRcaA

Natracare. (2021). *Natracare's organic cotton period products, including; tampons, applicator tampons, pads, curved panty liners* [Image]. https://unsplash.com/photos/r7UjnJHJxmY

Oziel Gómez. (2017). *Silhouette of hugging couple* [Image]. https://unsplash.com/photos/L8-0SAy-aoQ

Patrick Malleret. (2019). *Woman doing yoga pose* [Image]. https://unsplash.com/photos/p-v1DBkTrgo

Reproductive Health Supplies Coalition. (2019). *Emergency contraceptive pill* [Image]. https://unsplash.com/photos/RtRo-okGayk

Robina Weermeijer. (2019). *Human brain toy* [Image]. https://unsplash.com/photos/IHfOpAzzjHM

Smartworks Coworking. (2020). *Our coworking office space in Bangalore are conceptualized keeping in mind the needs of your growing business.* [Image]. https://unsplash.com/photos/cW4lLTavU80

Surface. (2023). *Woman in black and white* [Image]. https://unsplash.com/photos/E9NcsvbRVqo

Trnava University. (2022). *The Faculty of Health and Labor of the University of Trnava plans to launch a telemedicine simulation center soon.* https://unsplash.com/photos/1eBKFyZAnfA

2H Media. (2021). *Business & Work* [Image]. https://unsplash.com/photos/cdDDWLezAJ0

Vonecia Carswell. (2019). *Woman wearing yellow and white* [Image]. https://unsplash.com/photos/ZIab8W9KmmU

Windows. (2020). *Woman in blue long sleeve* [Images]. https://unsplash.com/photos/v94mlgvsza4